LIVING
WITH ILLNESS
OR DISABILITY

*10 Lessons of
Acceptance, Understanding,
and Perseverance*

SHARON A. GUTMAN, PHD, OTR/L

AOTA
PRESS
The American
Occupational Therapy
Association, Inc.

Vision Statement
AOTA advances occupational therapy as the pre-eminent profession in promoting the health, productivity, and quality of life of individuals and society through the therapeutic application of occupation.

Mission Statement
The American Occupational Therapy Association advances the quality, availability, use, and support of occupational therapy through standard-setting, advocacy, education, and research on behalf of its members and the public.

AOTA Staff
Frederick P. Somers, Executive Director
Christopher M. Bluhm, Chief Operating Officer
Audrey Rothstein, Director, Marketing and Communications

Chris Davis, Managing Editor, AOTA Press
Barbara Dickson, Production Editor

Robert A. Sacheli, Manager, Creative Services
Sarah E. Ely, Book Production Coordinator

Marge Wasson, Marketing Manager
Elizabeth Sarcia, Marketing Specialist

The American Occupational Therapy Association, Inc.
4720 Montgomery Lane
Bethesda, MD 20814
Phone: 301-652-AOTA (2682)
TDD: 800-377-8555
Fax: 301-652-7711
www.aota.org
To order: 1-877-404-AOTA (2682)

Disclaimers
This publication is designed to provide accurate and authoritative information in regard to the subject matter covered. It is sold or distributed with the understanding that the publisher is not engaged in rendering legal, accounting, or other professional service. If legal advice or other expert assistance is required, the services of a competent professional person should be sought.
—*From the Declaration of Principles jointly adopted by the American Bar Association and a Committee of Publishers and Associations*

It is the objective of the American Occupational Therapy Association to be a forum for free expression and interchange of ideas. The opinions expressed by the author of this work are her own and not necessarily those of the American Occupational Therapy Association.

ISBN: 1-56900-211-8

Library of Congress Control Number: 2005921807

Design by Sarah E. Ely
Composition by Electronic Quill, Silver Spring, MD
Printed by Edwards Brothers, Inc.

6/6/06

CONTENTS

Introduction   vii

Chapter 1   Marking the End of Grieving
for Our Old Life   1

Chapter 2   Accepting Ourselves and Our
Experience of Illness   17

Chapter 3   Learning Compassion and Forgiveness
for Ourselves and Others   31

Chapter 4   Accepting Life as It Unfolds and
Letting Go of Expectations   47

Chapter 5   Learning to Be Present in and
Appreciate the Moment   61

Chapter 6   Transforming Negativity Into Positive
Emotions and Actions   75

Chapter 7   Understanding and Letting Go of the
Illusion of Control   93

Chapter 8   Perceiving Life as a Spiritual Journey
and Understanding Illness as Part
of That Journey   107

Chapter 9   Finding the Gift in Our Experience and
Listening to the Messages of Illness   125

Chapter 10 Using What We've Learned to Help
Others and to Heal Ourselves 147

Further Reading 163

Index 167

About the Author 173

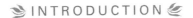

As an occupational therapist I've been afforded the opportunity to work with many people having an illness or disability. Many of the patients I've treated experienced serious injuries—such as spinal cord and traumatic brain injury— injuries that in my eyes left significant impairment in daily life. Over the years I have observed that some people— regardless of severe impairment—seemed to fare well and even prosper despite the enormous challenges of their illness or disability. These people were somehow able to repair their spirit and rebuild lives of personal satisfaction, while others appeared to lose hope and deteriorate. Throughout my practice I have continued to wonder what marked the difference between people who survived and even transformed their lives as a result of illness or disability and people who seemed to wither like twigs under the weight of a heavy snowfall. Was it resources and social support that marked the difference between those who thrived and those who could not regain their motivation to continue? Some of my patients with the most severe injuries had little resources or social and family supports. Yet they were grateful for the opportunity to be alive. Some even stated that they believed that their injury caused their lives to become more personally meaningful, as it enhanced their appreciation of the good they found within their days.

Then, in the year that my father retired he became ill—an unexpected event that jolted our family, as this was a man who had never been sick a day in his life. The initial diagnosis was thyroid cancer, but over the next eight years, his cancer spread through the lymphatic system to his abdomen, colon, and liver. The physical changes in his health were dramatic and swift. But what surpassed the changes in his physical status were the even greater changes in his personality.

My father had always been a stoic man for whom emotions were not a comfortable part of life. On occasion my family witnessed his laughter and sardonic sense of humor. More often, we were at the other end of his anger—anger that had likely smoldered over the years from growing up poor through the Depression and struggling financially to support himself and a family. My father was not an easy man to know, always holding his emotions at a distance. He had learned from an early age to become extremely independent and was not accustomed to asking for or accepting help. The idea that one should treat himself and others with compassion and gentleness was as alien to him as the moon. He had learned to be hard-nosed and tough-skinned to succeed in life—and materially he did succeed, which likely reinforced his belief that life demanded a hardened demeanor.

But over the course of his illness he changed, almost as if he had become another person. My father—who was acutely aware that his cancer was terminal—came to cherish life in a way that I had never seen from him. He became emotionally expressive and made certain that we knew how much he loved us. He became accepting of others, when before his illness almost everything and everyone served to disturb him. I was amazed when I witnessed acts of compassion from this man, not just to me, but to people he once disliked. He even began to speak of believing in a deeper meaning of life, after proclaiming to be an atheist for most of his adulthood. Even his style of speaking had changed from cynicism and negativity to optimism and encouragement. In the last years of his illness, when he had become physically incapacitated, he learned to accept help from those who loved him most—something he had never wanted or even allowed before his illness. Now, he was able to receive help with so much genuine gratitude that it was difficult to believe that he ever had trouble accepting assistance. The changes in his personality were so profound that I knew that he had been transformed in some way—some very positive way—by his illness.

I started recognizing common characteristics between my father's illness-induced transformation and that of my patients.' Over the years I met patients, colleagues, students, and friends who seemed inspired by their illness or disability experience to reconstruct their lives in very meaningful and healthy ways. Several years after my father's death I decided to interview these people to understand how illness or disability changed them and transformed their own lives and perspectives. As an occupational therapist I wanted to know if I could somehow use what they had discovered to help my own patients who—for whatever reasons—were unable to let go of the anger and sadness they felt as a result of illness or disability. When I began the interviews, one person would lead me to another who, they believed, had an even more amazing story. The people I interviewed for this book seemed to emerge effortlessly in my life as though they were meant to tell their story at this particular time. While all of the narratives are true and based on the real-life experiences of the people interviewed, all names and identifying information have been changed to protect the confidentiality and anonymity of those who generously contributed their stories.

Fifteen people were interviewed for this book, although portions of only 10 interviews were chosen for inclusion, as these best described transformational experiences. Ten common themes emerged throughout the interviews. These themes can be referred to as insights or lessons—those that people experienced as a result of living with illness or disability and having to reconstruct their daily lives to create meaning and value:

✍ 1. The need to grieve for one's pre-illness life to move on and to rebuild a meaningful life in the present

✍ 2. The need to accept oneself and one's illness to heal emotionally and to accept the idea that something good may come from illness that cannot be seen presently

✍ 3. The need to become more compassionate with oneself and others to promote health and to forgive oneself and others of past and present grievances to release the bitterness and anger that may impede health

✍ 4. The need to accept the way life unfolded instead of holding on to unrealistic expectations and feeling disappointed

✍ 5. The need to learn to experience and appreciate the present moment fully instead of worrying about the future or regretting the past

✍ 6. The need to change negative thoughts and emotions to positive ones that can help maintain a positive outlook

✍ 7. The need to let go of attempts to control life and to recognize what can and cannot be realistically controlled

✍ 8. The belief that life is a spiritual journey and that illness or disability is part of that journey—that both may bring life lessons that are painful but valuable

✍ 9. The belief that illness or disability may be a message to adopt more healthy emotional and physical behaviors and that the messages of both may be akin to hidden gifts that cannot be presently understood

🍂 10. The need to use what has been learned through illness or disability to help others to ultimately heal oneself.

While each of these 10 insights or lessons appear simple, they are often difficult to integrate into daily practice and commonly require some time before they become ingrained into one's life perspective—before they become second nature and no longer need to be consciously thought of to enact. The people interviewed in this book frequently expressed that they still struggle with the practice of many of the insights, finding that, to benefit from such wisdom, they must apply the insights daily. In this respect, the lessons become a life practice—a way of living. These 10 lessons do not seem to emerge in any particular order or even in a linear progression. Rather, people struggle with each at different times throughout the course of their illness or disability. Some insights occur simultaneously, some in tandem. The one common feature is that they have to be practiced consistently for individuals to receive their benefits.

This book describes the 10 insights or lessons of people who have been able to use what they have learned from illness or disability to rebuild their lives into meaningful existences marked by accomplishment, contentment, helping others, and finding simple joys. There are 10 chapters in this book—each describing one of the insights or lessons. Each offers one individual's narrative, recounting how that insight became a prominent part of his or her life perspective as a result of illness or disability. Each chapter also includes exercises that will help readers incorporate the insights into daily life to enhance life meaning and satisfaction. These exercises infuse occupational therapy practice with Eastern techniques and Western cognitive therapy. The book can be used by therapists and clients working together or directly by individuals who wish to engage in their own self-exploration.

All human life is eventually touched by adversity and loss, whether it comes in the form of trauma or illness. And all illness walks hand in hand with loss. No human life escapes pain in one form or another. We can benefit from understanding how others have used the life wisdom they gained through the experience of illness or disability to transform their lives into ones that hold meaning and touch others in positive ways.

—**Sharon A. Gutman, PhD, OTR/L**
Associate Professor,
Occupational Therapy Program
Richard Stockton College
Pomona, New Jersey

ONE

MARKING THE END
OF GRIEVING FOR
OUR OLD LIFE

When people experience a life-altering illness or disability, many grieve for lost lifestyles, lost roles, and the lost identity of being a person without major health concerns. Grieving is part of the natural response to events that bring loss, and individuals who do not mourn their losses sufficiently—and those who are unable to end their grieving—often experience difficulty adjusting to illness. Although grieving is part of the natural process of healing, one must release the attachment to one's life before illness to create quality and satisfaction in one's present life.

The people interviewed for this book, who were able to transform their lives through illness or disability, described a time when they realized that, to build a new life, they had to stop grieving for their old life. They had to relinquish their past self-identity and much of what was familiar and comfortable in their world to be able to create a new life—one that would encompass illness or disability in such a way that life could still be livable on a daily basis.

Michael's Story About Grieving

I met Michael when he was a 41-year-old psychologist primarily counseling people who had experienced a traumatic accident or illness resulting in a life-altering disability. Michael's understanding of such life crises came first hand; at age 15, he sustained a head injury and partial paralysis in a motorcycle accident.

I REMEMBER BEING CAREFREE AT 15, or at least carefree the way I remember it now. It was summer, and I was enjoying my freedom from school for at least another month before going back. Sometimes in the early evening, when it was still light outside but the traffic had died down after rush hour, my father would let me ride his motorcycle around the block—just around the block, no farther.

In those days I was a typical headstrong teenager, all-American jock, cocky, ready to test my wings outside of my safe neighborhood in the 'burbs. Sometimes when my father wasn't around, I would sneak his bike out and take my friends for rides on it. So one day, when my father wasn't home, I took the bike out and insisted that my neighbor, who was a couple of years younger than me, come along for a ride. I'm not completely sure what happened next. We were at a stop sign—it was a four-way stop. I remember coming to a complete stop and seeing a lady in a car coming down the street. I guess I assumed that she would stop, so I started going, but she blew the stop sign and hit us. It was months later in the hospital when they told me what had happened and that my friend didn't make it.

They told me I was in a coma for four months. When I woke up, I remember trying to talk, and everything that came out was just gibberish. Both of my legs and my right arm were paralyzed. And I had damaged my brain so severely that for a very long time I had major cognitive problems. I had no short-term memory for at least a year, and I still have difficulty with my memory unless I write everything down. But when this first happened I was in complete denial. I didn't think there was anything wrong with me; I just wanted to go home and get back to my life. I kept thinking that school was going to start, and I had to be at football practice or I'd be cut from the team. That was all I cared about—making sure I wasn't cut from the team. My friends would sometimes come to the hospital, and they'd have such a sad look on their faces, and I could never figure out why. It was months before I really began to understand the limitations I faced. Maybe that was a good thing—not understanding the enormity of what had happened to me. Otherwise, I might have given up.

But after several months in the rehab hospital I was able to go home, and that's when I truly began to understand how my life had changed—and that it would never be the same again. I had missed a year of school, and when I went back I wasn't the same person as before. Everyone knew me as a jock—an athlete. I had a reputation for getting into one too many fights and winning them, and I was proud of the tough-guy image I had built. And dating, well, I was 15 when the accident happened, and my hormones were raging. I didn't have any problem having a good time with girls. When I think back, it just all seemed so easy then.

So anyway, here I am with this head injury—that was still pretty severe—and I'm in a wheelchair, and my speech is slurred. I think I had gained about 20, maybe 25 pounds since the injury. It was like Michael had gone away, and this alien had entered my life. But this alien was me. Inside I felt the same, even though everyone treated me differently and I couldn't do half the things in my life that I used to. Forget being on the football team, forget getting a driver's license—they said that maybe I'd be able to eventually learn how to drive an adapted car. Forget girls. Now the girls I knew just felt sorry for me. And now I had to have tutors to get me through remedial courses so that I could graduate from high school.

You know, at first, before I started back at school, I was really determined to get on with my life, and I had this expectation that I'd just start back at high school and pick up where I left off. It wasn't until I was at school that I realized how unrealistic this was. And when I started seeing how everyone was treating me, and how many things I needed help with, it just really hit me terribly, and I became very depressed.

I guess this is when I started grieving for my old life. I just wanted to be that carefree kid who had everything going for him. I wished so much that I could turn back the hands of time and change that one stupid decision to take my father's bike out. And on top of all of this, at some point it hit me, too, that I was responsible for my friend's death.

So I was grieving for my lost life and for this young boy who, because of my poor judgment, would never have the opportunity to live out his life. It was truly an awful, terribly lonely, bleak period in my life. There were really times that I didn't want to go on. I think that my father helped me the most with this. I would cry to him, "Dad, I don't know how to go on. I'll never have the kind of life I want. I can't walk, I can't think the way I used to." And he'd say, "Michael, you're OK. You didn't die in the accident. You're here for a reason. It's not going to be as easy as it used to be. Some things are just gonna come a little harder from now on. But you have to make the best of each day and find the thing that makes your life worth living." And that's when I realized that I had to give up my attachment to my old way of life and the expectations I had had for myself. I had to let go of the person I had been for 15 years and create a new life. And I slowly came to understand that this would be my challenge for the next years and that, eventually, this was what I wanted to help others do in the same situation.

I remember that I had seen an orthopedic surgeon who said that he could fix both of my hips, because I couldn't move them after the accident. And I was really hopeful that if I could just walk again, everything would go back to being the way it had been—and, of course, that I would be the same way I was before the accident. I had unrealistically put all of my hopes into this one surgery and into the idea of walking again. A team of specialists looked at my x-rays and said that they didn't recommend performing the surgery because there was bone growth around the femoral arteries and because there was a good chance that during the surgery the femoral arteries could be cut, leaving me completely paralyzed. I was really heartbroken. I thought that I had an opportunity to get rid of my disability, and I couldn't.

After that I disciplined myself to be more accepting of myself and to live with what I had. I began to make a concerted effort to concentrate on what I *could* do instead of focusing on my limitations. I would coach myself with self-talk. I would talk to myself all day long, cheering myself to keep going and to appreciate what was good in each day. And I stopped punishing myself because of the accident—because I had made a bad decision to take out the motorcycle when I shouldn't have.

I can't change the past. I can't change the fact that I rode the motorcycle with my neighbor on the back and a lady blew a stop sign and crashed into us. I stopped grieving for the past when I realized that I couldn't change what had happened to me, but that I *could* influence the kind of life I was having in the present. I remember that at some point, I consciously decided to stop grieving for my old identity—to let it go and create a new life that would be meaningful to me on a day-to-day basis. After what I went through—and survived—I knew that I wanted to help other people who found themselves in the same place I did as a 15-year-old kid. And that wasn't easy either.

The whole journey has been a real struggle and sometimes still is. But I was determined to persevere and find a way to reach my goal, no matter what. After my accident it took me three more years to complete high school, five years to complete undergraduate school, and another five years to get my counseling degree. There were times when I just wanted to give up—when the obstacles and barriers seemed too overwhelming. But I also knew that I didn't have a choice. It was either give up and let a bad decision I made as a teenager ruin the rest of my life, or turn my life into something I could be proud of. And that always kept me motivated to keep going when I was ready to quit—that I wanted my life to be something I could be proud of.

I received my counseling degree about 10 years ago and built my practice helping people of all ages start life anew after experiencing some trauma or illness that left them with a severe disability. So I feel that I've come full circle, so to speak. And when I look back, sure, I wish that the accident had never happened, but it *did* happen. And I could have allowed it to change my life in a very bad way. I didn't want to do that. I wanted to be able to look back and see how the accident led me to a place in my life where I'm proud of the work I'm doing with others. And I can honestly say today that I'm proud of what I've been through and what I survived, and I'm proud of who I am.

Exercise 1: Recognizing the Cyclic Nature of Life and Events

One of the first steps in the grieving process involves the recognition that human life is characterized by cycles involving natural rhythms of ups and downs, of gentle and challenging periods—much like the tides and the seasons. Every human being experiences both success and failure and periods of ease and struggle. Life teaches us that these natural cycles occur no matter how much we try to fend them off or protect ourselves from adversity. Nevertheless, we tend to expect our lives to be untouched by difficulty, and we are often caught off guard when hardship strikes. One of the greatest tools that can ease our passage through periods of challenge is the understanding—and conscious remembrance—that hardship is a natural part of human life and will eventually, if we persevere, be followed by a period of greater ease and comfort. This insight can help anchor our lives when crisis hits and we fear that life will never return to its once-peaceful course.

One of the first steps in ending the grieving process is to recognize the cyclic nature of life and to remember that the cycle we are now experiencing will one day be replaced by another, and later still by another. If we are experiencing crisis, we must remember that greater peace will eventually follow; if we are experiencing relative calmness, we must be conscious that a cycle of greater turmoil will likely enter our lives to bring new challenges that promote growth.

Chronicle the major cycles in your life by drawing a timeline and recording periods of crisis and peacefulness. For each cycle, describe

🌿 What qualities made the period difficult or easy?

🌿 What did you learn from each cycle, and how did the cycle contribute to your personal growth? How did you change as a result of experiencing that cycle?

🌿 How did that cycle contribute to forming the personality that you have today?

🌿 Make sure that you include all the major life cycles, particularly the good ones. In times of crisis, our perspective tends to become negative, and that negative lens colors how we remember our past. People experiencing conflict tend to remember periods of greater difficulty more readily than periods of calm.

Exercise 2: Allowing Ourselves to Grieve

The Taoists have a saying, "The only way out is through." (See "Further Reading" for more resources on Taoism.) When one experiences a major life illness—particularly of a chronic nature—a grieving process becomes necessary to release one's attachment to the goals, expectations, and satisfactions of life before illness. To rebuild a life that is meaningful—despite the illness—one must grieve for the lifestyle that one was forced, beyond one's control, to relinquish.

In Western society, people often don't allow themselves either the opportunity or sufficient time to grieve their losses. The grieving process is usually experienced in the context of the death of a person, but symbolic or nontangible deaths—such as the loss of a cherished friendship or the loss of a pre-illness lifestyle—must be grieved, too, if a rebirth is to be experienced. Sometimes people do not allow themselves the opportunity to grieve because they want to be strong for others or believe that a demonstration of emotion will be perceived as a sign of weakness. As children we may have learned that grieving is self-indulgent or a luxury for those who have to struggle to provide materially for themselves and others. We may have been chastised for "feeling sorry for ourselves" or chided to "snap out of it."

Examine your ideas about the grieving process. Ask yourself these questions, and record your answers in a journal:

❧ From whom did you first gain your ideas about the grieving process? From parents, older relatives, religious figures?

❧ What did you learn from them about the proper way to grieve? How did they grieve? Did they express their emotions freely, or hold them inside? How long did they allow themselves to grieve? Did their grieving process take only a few short days? Or did it seem too long to you or to other family members?

❧ What types of events were grieved in your family? Some families allow a grieving process to occur only in response to death. Were there other events, besides death, that were grieved by your family members?

❧ What are your feelings about grieving? Do you feel that it's self-indulgent? Or that you have to be strong for your loved ones?

❧ Do you feel entitled to grieve for the loss of your identity as a person without illness?

In the grieving process, it is important to feel our emotions—such as sadness and anger—fully. One way to emerge from unsettling feelings of sadness and anger is to experience such emotions in their entirety. Suppressing feelings by suffocating them with other experiences (such as alcohol, pain medication, food, or sex) will not offer the opportunity to work through and eventually release these emotions. To end the grieving process and rebuild our lives, it is important to thoroughly acknowledge the feelings of sadness and anger we hold about our illness.

Identify the three most meaningful things that you were forced to give up as a result of illness, and record these in your journal. Describe why the loss of each has caused sadness or anger for you. Be certain that you examine whether you truly had to forfeit these things, or whether they still can be part of your life in a modified form.

Talking with loved ones (or a special loved one) about your sadness and anger can be cathartic and can facilitate the grieving process. Sharing such feelings also builds intimacy and trust. Sometimes, however, we may fear that our loved one cannot assume the weight of these emotions. If this is the case, ask your loved one directly if he or she wants to hear your feelings and to share his or her own feelings. When emotions are kept bottled—particularly within the context of a relationship—they will emerge through unconscious actions or in angry outbursts that could be avoided by confronting these feelings directly. If you feel that you cannot express yourself orally, it may be helpful to write a letter to one or more loved ones in which you convey how your illness has caused you to experience sadness or anger.

Sometimes it is helpful to write a letter to yourself. You may write the letter from the perspective of the person you are today and address it to the person you were before you experienced illness in your life. Or you may address the letter to the person you hope to be a year from now.

Whether you communicate by talking to others or by writing letters to loved ones or to yourself, the goal is to express your feelings so that you can become aware of and eventually release them. One of the strongest impediments to rebuilding life is to remain stuck in an emotion that we cannot move past. Once we are aware of our emotions and have expressed them fully, the next step in dissolving their hold on our lives is to become involved in daily activities that provide joy and meaning, rather than allowing sadness and anger to prevent our continued participation in life.

Exercise 3: Recognizing When Our Grieving Process Is Almost Over

Allowing ourselves sufficient opportunity to grieve is important. Understanding when our grieving process is near an end—so that we can begin to move forward—is critical to our ability to maintain our spirit to live. Often when people are ready to end the grieving process, they begin to experience small inner urges to engage in an activity. The activity may be modest at first (such as getting out of bed) or more involved (planting flowers). Initially, such inner impulses to engage in life-renewing activity may be fleeting. However, the more we act on such impulses, the more often and intensely we feel them. When we act on them, such impulses grow like a wave building momentum as it nears the shore. The key is to watch for these urges and seize them. We can use them to pull ourselves out of periods of stillness, nonmovement, and inaction to periods of greater involvement in life.

In the past weeks, have you noticed any desire—even for a fleeting moment—to participate in an activity you once enjoyed? Or to finish a project that you had begun a while ago? What did you do with this urge? Was it too overwhelming to act on? Or did it seem unworthy of the energy required?

For the rest of the week, note when these urges occur. It may be helpful to record in your journal (1) the date and time, (2) whether the urge occurred in response to anything happening in your immediate environment, and (3) which activities you felt motivated to engage in. Record whether you acted on the impulse, and describe the feelings you had in response to it.

The next time you experience an impulse to become active in your life again, try to act on it—even in the smallest way—and observe how this feels. Praise yourself for the smallest act or effort. Do not expect too much of yourself; it is important to be realistic about which activities you truly have energy for. Do not berate yourself if an impulse comes and you do not act on it. Remember, everything occurs in its own time.

Exercise 4: Marking the End of Our Past Life With Rituals and Celebration

Many cultures use ritual and celebration to mark the transition from one life period to the next. Sometimes using a tangible event to identify a symbolic life transition can help us move through our life's journey. Once the grieving process for our pre-illness life has been completed, we may find it helpful to use ritual and celebration to mark the transition to a new life passage—signifying a rebirth.

Acknowledging the blessings of our pre-illness life with celebration and ritual can help us feel ready to transition into the next passage of life. Celebration and ritual can enable us to remember the gratitude we feel for the life we have been fortunate to lead. From the following activities, select those that are most personally meaningful and could help you mark the end of your grieving and begin a new life passage:

❧ In your journal, list the joys that have occurred in your life; chronicle your entire life, recording the things that you are thankful for. Do not forget to include both the modest and the seemingly trivial, as these are easy to overlook but can amount to much gratitude. When you are finished, consciously offer thanks for being blessed with this fortune. Ask that this next passage of your life be marked by life events that also will bring the opportunity for thankfulness.

❧ Choose a date marking the symbolic death of your pre-illness life and the rebirth of your new life passage. The date may be a diagnosis or when the symptoms first occurred. Or it may be when you decided to begin rebuilding your life in accordance with your own goals for meaning. Use candles and flowers to acknowledge this date, as you would any other traditional death or birth. Ask that your journey provide you with the opportunities to experience gratitude and joy in this new passage.

❧ Hold a small gathering for your intimate friends and loved ones in which you acknowledge the people and events in your life for which you have gratitude. Toast your life's joys and the events and people that have made your life valuable and full. This is an especially powerful ritual, because you are using the present moment to express gratitude to others. Ask that these people be part of the journey that you are now embarking on, and request their presence and assistance as you begin to travel on a new life path.

❧ Write thank you letters to your loved ones and intimate friends in which you articulate your gratitude for their friendship. Communicating your feelings of gratitude in written form can be healing, even if you do not send the letters. Letters also can be written to people who are no longer living or to people with whom you are no longer in contact; sometimes these are the most cathartic, as they offer us occasions to convey feelings we never had the opportunity to share.

❧ Maintain a gratitude journal, a daily journal in which you record the things that you are thankful for each day. A gratitude journal can help us maintain a balanced perspective when we are in the midst of crisis. It also can help us remember that all of human life is characterized by cycles of struggle and ease and that, even in times of pain, there are still occasions for which to be thankful.

Exercise 5: Creating a New Self-Image and Passages to a New Life

Before we can begin to think about creating a new life for ourselves, we must fully assess the life we have led up until the present moment.

✎ First, go back to the timeline of your life you drew in Exercise 1 and highlight all of the major life experiences that have been meaningful to you. For each event, indicate how it changed your life and shaped who you are today. Identify events that have given you joy and made you proud, as well as those that have saddened you.

✎ Are there gaps in your timeline created by events that you desired but that never transpired? How has the absence of these expected events changed the course of your life and shaped your personality?

✎ Have there been wonderful events that have occurred that you never expected? How have these changed your life course and shaped your personality?

Recording your major life events on a timeline and understanding how these events have contributed to your life course will help you gain a more balanced perspective of your life's journey as a whole. It is easy to focus on the negative when we are feeling unwell. When this occurs, it becomes necessary to reassess both the adversities and the gratifications of our lives to gain a more realistic perspective.

Now that you have compiled an overview of your entire life, it may be beneficial to visualize what you desire for this next life passage. If you could design the blueprints—while maintaining realistic expectations regarding your illness—what would this next passage of your life be like? Do you wish for greater intimacy with loved ones and friends? To contribute in some meaningful way to your community? To spend more time enjoying activities that are healing for your body, mind, and spirit? Are there specific goals that you want to accomplish?

View this next passage of your life as the next step of your journey. Answering these questions in writing will help you formulate the kind of passage you would like to create for yourself. Crystallize your thoughts about the following in writing to help you solidify both your mental conception of what life can be like and your commitment to your goals:

❧ Write a description about who you would like to become in this next phase of life. Think back to the kind of person you have been. How have others viewed you? Is there a difference between how others have viewed you and how you feel internally? Describe the kind of person that you would strive to become if you could set your journey's itinerary. What learning opportunities would you establish for yourself?

❧ Identify three specific ways in which you would like to grow personally. Identify methods, paths, or learning opportunities that could help you grow in the ways that you identified. It's most helpful to take small steps to achieve new goals. Choose one of the three goals that you have identified for your personal growth and identify two ways that you could begin to integrate this growth into your everyday life for the next three weeks. Each day, note the efforts that you make toward this one goal (it is helpful to record your experience in your journal). Do not ignore small efforts. Do not berate yourself for days in which you were unable to make any effort. Instead, praise yourself for each effort that you were able to make, no matter how minor it may seem.

Remember, the process of change requires much time and is characterized by natural gains and setbacks. Change usually occurs through perseverance and the accumulation of small attempts made over an extended period of time. Remember also that the process of change is just as important as the end result. Too often we lose this insight and devalue the attempts we make to reach a goal, particularly if we do not experience the end goal in the exact way in which we originally anticipated. Devaluing our effort only discourages future effort. Instead, we benefit by valuing all of our attempts to facilitate positive change, not only the end result. We also should be prepared to accept the fact that the end result will probably look very different from our initial expectations.

TWO

ACCEPTING OURSELVES AND OUR EXPERIENCE OF ILLNESS

There often comes a time in people's lives when they realize that, to live a life that is personally meaningful and satisfying, they must accept themselves as they are, with all of their inadequacies and self-judgments. In accepting themselves, people come to perceive themselves as lovable beings who might have made mistakes but who did the best they could. The people interviewed for this book reached a point in their lives when they no longer felt the need to grieve for an old self or for an ideal life free of illness or disability. In accepting themselves, they accepted their illness as well, viewing the illness not as an enemy but as an experience through which they were learning to live more meaningful lives. As people grew in self-acceptance, they became less influenced by external measures of success. The values of society became less important; they no longer measured their self-worth or judged their life's accomplishments against society's standards.

The people who transformed their lives through illness or disability also recognized that, in the natural course of human life, there will be good days and bad days. They learned to stop berating themselves for the bad days or begrudging the "lost time." Instead, all life situations, both affirming and difficult, became meaningful learning experiences—opportunities to grow and to share what they had learned with others. The difficult days allowed them to better appreciate the days that felt more comfortable.

Jim's Experience of Self-Acceptance

At 53, Jim had become a beloved and respected college professor whom students adored, confided in, and trusted. He was working in his college's Office of Special Education Services providing counseling for students with disabilities who required accommodations to complete their education. When Jim went to college, such services were not readily available to help him navigate the environmental barriers and attitudinal misconceptions he experienced in response to a movement disorder he acquired in childhood. When he was 6, Jim was sent home from school with the chicken pox, which later developed into encephalitis. The encephalitis was treated but left Jim with a movement disorder known as idiopathic torsion dystonia. *Idiopathic* means that the origin of the disorder is unknown; *torsion dystonia* means that the muscles of the body contract, producing twisting movements that result in abnormal body postures.

MY LITTLE BODY SEEMED TO POSSESS a mind of its own. I'd suddenly go into writhing positions or twist around, with my neck held back or my eyes held shut. And when this would happen, I couldn't move out of these positions—it was like being trapped in a body possessed. Before I was 10 I had had three major surgeries performed by a doctor who said that he had a new technique for curing such conditions.

I'm not really sure what he did, but he operated on my brain three times. The surgeries didn't seem to do much about my twisted posture, and it seemed as though I was losing more and more control in my legs and arms.

Between the uncontrollable twisting positions and the weakness in my legs and arms, I needed to use a wheelchair and a host of adaptive equipment. I also missed what seemed like years of school, which probably held me back both socially and academically. As you can imagine, all I wanted to do was have a life like my older brother, whom I idealized as normal. He had all of the friends and social activities that I craved; he went to school, he did homework, he played baseball, he could cut up his own food on his dinner plate. I must have lived vicariously through him for most of my childhood and adolescence.

When I wasn't recuperating from surgery, I went to a special school for children with disabilities. Many of these children were severely mentally challenged, and I continued to lack the normal stimulation that a child needs to develop. I felt very out of place in this setting. And I longed for the opportunities to go out into what I thought of as the real world. But when my parents took me to the park or took me and my brother to a restaurant, I felt like an animal at the zoo. People stared. Kids my age laughed or turned away. These were humiliating experiences, and I felt very ashamed and very bad about myself. When you're a child or teenager, all you want to do is fit in and be accepted by your peers. At times it was excruciating for me to be so different from everyone else. In fact, before I was in my 20s, I had never even met anyone else who shared my unique disorder. And this made me feel even more isolated and set apart.

Needless to say, I had great difficulty feeling comfortable in my own skin. I was naturally shy and introverted to begin with, and this just exacerbated my inability to make any real connection with anyone. I thought that people would immediately dislike me when they met me, so after years of being alone I gave up trying to make any friends. By the time I was a teenager I had developed a very strong dislike of myself. And of course I kept masochistically comparing myself to my brother who, as a teenager, seemed to me to have all of the graces and blessings of a chosen son—he was handsome, smart, athletic, sociable. And I was just his little brother who was cursed by God to have this incurable affliction. I grew up watching him lead the life I wanted.

We were raised Catholic, and for many years I was very angry at God for giving me this disease. As a child I was taught to believe that God gives people only what they can handle, and no more. And I kept thinking that there must be some special reason why God gave me this disease. But growing up I could never figure out what that reason was. And sometimes I felt that even God had rejected me. It took me many, many years before I realized that God didn't send this disease for me to suffer. And it took even longer to realize that I had rejected myself.

It wasn't until I went away to college and got involved in the disability rights movement that I started meeting people who grew up having the same experiences as me—people who had some disability that set them apart from the ordinary world and who as a result felt isolated, shamed, and unacceptable. And meeting these people was a revelation for me, because for the first time my experience was validated—it was the norm. I wasn't different anymore. I was young and vibrant and intelligent and capable—despite the disability I had. Finding this group of people—and being involved in the effort to secure equal rights for people with disabilities—was the first time in my life that I felt acceptance from

others, and that allowed me to start feeling greater acceptance for myself.

Meeting my wife also helped me to feel that I was lovable. And it was the first time that I ever experienced a deep
sense of love for another person. Feeling that amount of love
for another human being makes you realize that, if you can
feel that much love for someone, then there must be a part of
you that is good and loving, too. That if you can feel that
degree of love for another, then that ability to love must
mean that you are lovable as well. I met my wife at college
when we were both working on increasing access to public
buildings for people using wheelchairs. My wife was born
with cerebral palsy and had experienced many of the same
prejudices and stereotypes that I did growing up. People
judged her to be mentally impaired, even though she has
always been highly intelligent. She taught me a lot about
self-acceptance and believing in your own worth—despite
the subtle and not-so-subtle messages from other people that
you're really just an inconvenience.

I got my doctorate in education in school counseling and
have always been lucky enough to work at universities that
have valued diversity and have given me the opportunity to
teach about how our society deals with disability. And in the
last decade I've been fortunate to head my university's Office
of Special Education Services. This has been the greatest job
for me because it's allowed me to help students get a college
education without all of the barriers and misconceptions about
disability that I endured. And it's allowed me to help some of
these kids start accepting themselves a little more.

When I think about myself today, I don't think of someone who's disabled. I have limitations and challenges just like
everybody else. I've realized that everyone has some type of
personal challenge that they must face and deal with in life.

But my disability doesn't stand out in my mind anymore; I don't define myself by my disability the way I used to. In fact, I think today I have more acceptance for myself than at any other time in my life. I've been through a lot, and I know that I can survive and that I have inner strength. I feel very comfortable with myself and very good about the person I've become and what I've done with my life.

One of the blessings that my experience of disability has given me is the greater ability to be accepting of others. I clearly remember what it was like to want people to be more accepting of me—to be able to see me and not just my physical disability. And to be able to separate me—the core of who I am—from the disability they saw on the surface. My experience of disability has allowed me to look past someone's limitations and see the loving, intelligent person that is there. It's easy for me to empathize with people who are different, because for so many years I felt different from everyone. For so many of my years I felt that people judged me only by what they saw on the outside. And so now, when I meet a student or anyone with some kind of disability, I try to make a connection with that person's inner self—I want them to know that I see them as a capable, lovable, intelligent person. And it's that person whom I build a relationship with—not with their disability. I treat people with as much respect and with as much acceptance as I have in my heart to give. And I have a great deal of acceptance in my heart today—it's grown as I've learned to accept myself.

Exercise 1: Exploring Our Ideas About Acceptance

One of the most difficult practices to achieve is *self-acceptance*—accepting everything about ourselves, including personality traits and psychological aspects that we may have unconsciously disowned. To begin to practice self-acceptance, it is important to first identify those things about ourselves that we know we have difficulty accepting.

🖊 Make a list of the things about yourself that you find difficult to accept, and next to each item, indicate why you think this part of yourself is unacceptable.

🖊 Ask yourself if other people have found this quality to be unsatisfactory. If your answer is yes, was there a specific person (or persons) who made you feel this way?

🖊 As you were growing up, how did you learn about acceptance? Were your family members accepting of each other? Were they able to accept themselves?

🖊 What did you learn about acceptance from religious figures, schoolteachers, and friends?

🖊 Growing up, did you learn that accepting yourself was an important component of emotional well-being?

🖊 Has there been anyone in your life whom you felt completely accepted by? If so, how did this feel to you?

We often learn from religious figures and schoolteachers that it is important to accept others; however, we rarely learn how to accept ourselves. If this is true for you, try to imagine that the qualities that you find unacceptable in yourself now belong to another person—choose someone you care a great deal about. Is it easier for you to accept these traits in another person than in yourself? If so, imagine loving this person even with those unacceptable characteristics. Can you imagine extending that same love you feel for this person to yourself? Practice offering to yourself the same acceptance you have of this person. Many of the people interviewed for this book stated that they were able to learn self-acceptance after they recognized that they accepted their own unacceptable qualities in the people they cared for most.

Exercise 2: Practicing Mindfulness Training

Mindfulness training is a Buddhist practice in which one disciplines one's mind to identify and challenge specific beliefs and old thought patterns that do not support emotional well-being. (See "Further Reading" for more resources on Buddhism.) Often thoughts we do not realize we have run rampant in our minds and then negatively influence our well-being and ability to adjust to life circumstances. To accept ourselves, we must first become aware of the unconscious stream of negative thoughts that influence our emotional and physical health.

First, practice catching your thoughts and consciously identifying them. Write down the flow of thoughts that come into your mind in the course of 15 minutes. Continue to practice this until you become more adept at recognizing the thoughts that enter your mind throughout the day. Truly becoming conscious of one's daily thoughts commonly requires disciplined practice over many months.

Often our thoughts about ourselves are overly critical—for example, "I'm no good," "No one really cares about me," "No one would appreciate the skills I have," or "No one cares that I'm sick." Practice catching yourself when you begin to experience thoughts that you or certain personal qualities are unacceptable. When you have these thoughts, stop what you're doing and record them in a journal. Indicate the time of day and whether a specific situation elicited these thoughts. Maintaining a daily journal can help us become aware of our overly critical thinking patterns and end their influence on our daily emotional well-being.

Then challenge the validity of each negative thought. Ask yourself if each thought is truly accurate. Is it true that no one really cares about you? Or that you have no talents that others would appreciate? For each negative thought about feeling unacceptable, list the facts of your life that challenge the validity of that thought.

Your goal is to reach the point at which you can consciously catch all negative thoughts as they occur and counteract them with more positive—yet still realistic— thoughts. For example, when you catch the thought "No one really cares that I'm sick," you might challenge it with the thought "There are several people in my life who have expressed concern and who have offered help. I may not have had the courage to ask for their assistance." When you catch the thought "I have no talents that others would appreciate," you might counteract this belief with the thought "I have several talents that I have not shared with many others. Others may value my skills if I have the courage to share them. I may try to share my talents with a few chosen others to see their reaction."

It is frequently helpful to share negative thoughts with a therapist or trusted confidant who can help you challenge the validity of these thoughts. Often, we need the realistic feedback of others when our own thoughts have become distorted by sadness, hopelessness, or depression. We often do not recognize the extent to which our thoughts have become distorted, and the realistic feedback of a therapist or someone who cares about us can help us effectively change our negative thought processes.

Exercise 3: Accepting That We Are Doing the Best That We Can

Sometimes we feel that we are not measuring up to our own standards. We berate ourselves unnecessarily for perceived failures or weaknesses. When we do this, we are indeed our own worst enemy. What if we learned to be our own best friend—our own coach, cheering on our victories? What if we learned to appreciate that we are doing the best we can with the resources we have available? These steps can assist you in this process:

𝕀 Using mindfulness training, catch those instances when you are berating yourself for self-perceived failures, weaknesses, or mistakes. Identify in your journal what you are reprimanding yourself for and why.

𝕀 Identify whether anyone else elicited your feelings of failure or weakness, both in the present moment and in the past while you were growing up.

𝕀 Recognize the expectations you held for yourself in the situations you identified. How did you originally form these expectations? Did you learn them from others (family members, religious figures, schoolteachers, friends)? When did you take on these expectations as your own? If you assumed these expectations in your formative years (child-hood and adolescence), do you still wish to hold these expec-tations as an adult? Do they serve your emotional well-being as an adult?

Imagine that a loving mentor, teacher, or coach has observed the same situation for which you are presently rebuking yourself. Imagine that this mentor acknowledges that you did the best you could at the time and honors what you were truly able to accomplish in the situation. Imagine that this mentor helps you understand that the goal you are seeking involves a process that requires time and sustained effort. Imagine also that this teacher helps you appreciate what you did accomplish and expresses faith in your ability to reach your goal. Most of all, imagine that this teacher accepts your efforts as valuable and helps you accept them as well.

Now, instead of perceiving the situation as a failure, reconsider it as part of the process needed to achieve your goal. Recognize what you were able to accomplish, and acknowledge its contribution to your personal growth. Identify what you learned from this experience that will help you eventually achieve your goal (or revised goal). Record these insights in your journal for later review:

☙ Determine whether your initial goal requires revision. Often, when our original plans do not flow smoothly, modifying those plans enables us to reach our goals through another route. Sometimes, too, modifying the original goal helps us achieve similar but different success experiences that still provide meaning and satisfaction that we could not initially have foreseen.

☙ Repeat this practice every time you catch yourself criticizing your efforts because of some perceived failure. Repeat these steps until you become adept at replacing your perceptions of failed experience with acceptance of the effort you put forth. Practicing these skills daily will help you value your effort as part of the larger process of growth and learning that takes place in all human lives.

As with all effort to change self-berating thoughts to more self-accepting thoughts, it is often helpful to practice these techniques with a therapist or trusted confidant who can help you see when you are unjustly harsh on yourself or are being overly critical.

Exercise 4: Changing the Way We Think About Our Illness or Disability

One very important characteristic of people who transform their lives through illness or disability is their ability to accept it—and thus to accept themselves fully. Accepting illness or disability is particularly difficult within a society and medical culture that view illness and disability as enemies that must be combated or conquered.

It is first important to explore your own views about illness and disability:

❧ Write down all of the ideas you hold about illness and disability. Do you view them as an enemy that must be destroyed? As a punishment from God or a test of faith? As a random, senseless occurrence without meaning?

❧ Where do your ideas about illness and disability come from? Think back to your childhood and memories of people you knew who had an illness. How did your family view that person's illness? What did that person believe about his or her illness? What were the views of the religious figures, schoolteachers, and peers in your life? Did any of these views influence how you perceive your own illness or disability?

❧ Instead of perceiving your illness or disability as an enemy (or a punishment, a test of faith, a random occurrence), think about what you have learned from this experience that you would not have otherwise learned. What has it taught you that has been positive in your life? For example, has it taught you strength or independence? Has it made you become more compassionate or accepting of others? Has it taught you how to receive help from others? Has it provided opportunities for you to help others? Record your insights in your journal.

❧ Periodically ask yourself this question, "What is my illness teaching me?"

Being able to accept one's illness or disability often depends on one's ability to acknowledge and value the positive things that have come out of the experience. It is said that our greatest challenges often provide our greatest lessons, and out of life crisis comes opportunity. Although no one desires disease or impairment, it is easier to accept if we are able to find the good that can emerge from adversity.

One of the most effective ways to learn self-acceptance is to join a group whose members offer genuine acceptance. Some people find help in a support group in which people experiencing the same life crisis come together for emotional support and education about available resources. Others benefit from joining a religious or spiritual group whose members practice acceptance to help them learn greater self-acceptance. When we feel accepted by trusted, valued others, we can often transfer that acceptance to ourselves.

The danger in depending on a group to learn self-acceptance occurs when the group dissolves and we no longer feel acceptable without that external support. In such cases, we have not truly learned self-acceptance but rather have come to rely on an external source for something we need to give to ourselves. Joining a group that practices acceptance is but one way of many to facilitate self-acceptance, and we need to use other methods as well.

Working with a skilled therapist who demonstrates acceptance also can be effective. A therapist can both challenge ideas that we are unacceptable and help us practice skills that enhance our own self-acceptance.

THREE

LEARNING COMPASSION AND FORGIVENESS FOR OURSELVES AND OTHERS

When people who had transformed their lives through illness or disability began to accept themselves and that illness or disability, they became more compassionate with both themselves and others; their awareness that they are worthwhile beings who desire to be treated with kindness grew. But rather than deflecting the responsibility of caring for themselves onto others, they understood that it was they who must first learn to be compassionate with themselves and to treat themselves with kindness—to be gentle with themselves as the course of their illness and their life journey unfolded. Such compassion became a daily practice.

In turn, as they learned to express compassion for themselves, they also learned to extend that compassion to others. Through their own challenges and adversity, people become better able to understand the pain of others. And in better understanding the pain of others, they come to realize that all human suffering is the same; no one person's pain is any less significant than any other's. All individuals deserve to be treated compassionately.

The act of compassion walks alongside the act of forgiveness. When people begin to view themselves and their struggles with compassion, they are able to be more forgiving of themselves as well. They recognize that mistakes are part of the lessons learned in life, and they stop berating themselves for perceived infractions or lost opportunities. They make peace with themselves and with others, recognizing that conflict unsettles the healing process and that, in comparison to the life challenges they are facing or have faced, petty conflicts with others do not matter. When people are able to make peace with themselves, they bring peace to their lives.

Sue's Story About Learning Compassion

Sue was a 42-year-old elementary school teacher who appeared to have an endless supply of energy, enthusiasm, and gentleness for her spirited group of 4th graders. But there were periods in Sue's life when she had neither the energy nor the desire to get out of bed in the morning and the thought of getting dressed seemed an overwhelming task that required more effort than she was capable of giving. Sue had lived with chronic recurrent depression since her early 20s, when she experienced her first major depressive episode.

AS A CHILD I WAS WHAT YOU'D CALL dysthymic or melancholic. I was a sensitive child and introverted, shy. I was happy to be left alone with my art supplies. I think that I was a sad child, for no apparent reason when I think back. It's not like I came from an abusive home or suffered great losses in childhood. In fact, I probably had much more than most: loving parents who were responsible and took care of me, a beautiful neighborhood to grow up in, the best public schools in the area. But there was always something different about me, something that was different from the other children in my elementary school classes. I was never carefree like them. I could never give myself to play and fantasy with abandon the way they seemed to. My teachers called me conscientious and serious. Yes, that's it; I was always a bit too serious, like I had the weight of the world's problems on my shoulders at age 6. And even at 6—and all the while growing up—I always felt like I had the soul of a 90-year-old. My soul was old from childhood rather than carefree as a child's should be.

When I was 13 and hit puberty, my emotions became a little more stormy. It's not that I had problems in school; on the contrary, I was the perfect student—academically gifted, responsible, and polite. But at 13 I think I stopped smiling for a very long time. I'm not sure that I smiled through the rest of my adolescence until maybe 18. I felt very sad inside, and at the time I didn't understand it. And of course my parents thought that this was typical behavior for a teenager. None of us understood that this melancholy was a precursor of later depression. There were no signs other than the sadness that was almost always with me. And I guess that no one picked it up because I had learned over the years to fit in by hiding how I truly felt inside. So I became pretty adept at projecting the image that I was OK. You know, "smile, Sue"—so many people would say this to me that I just started smiling to stop them from probing further. I could keep up this facade for about 15 minutes, and then I had to excuse myself before the facade fell apart.

At 24 I experienced my first severe depression. I had just finished college and couldn't find a job. My boyfriend had broken up with me, and I had moved back home with my parents because I couldn't support myself. It was like I was sliding downward and couldn't pull myself back up. I felt like a failure. I had graduated in the top 10 percent of my class, and now I couldn't get a job. My parents kept pushing me to get married, and I started feeling that there was something wrong with me because I couldn't find work, because I wasn't married, because I was an adult living at home.

I don't really remember how it happened now, except that one day I woke up and no longer wanted to be alive. And every day it got worse. In the morning I would awake with extreme anxiety and agitation, as though I was in a life-threatening situation. I just wanted to get out, but there was nowhere to go. I had no appetite and lost 15 pounds, going from 103 to 88 lbs. I didn't want to do anything or see anyone. All of my past interests meant nothing to me. There's a term, *anhedonia*, which means the inability to experience joy, and that's exactly what I felt. I walked around all day with this horrible sense of dread and anguish, and I wished that I were dead—that I could be released from this torture through death. In fact, I had my suicide all planned out, although I never acted on any of those thoughts. But for three months straight—with no relief—I walked around all day in this state.

And if I was tortured you can just imagine how my parents felt. They had no idea what was happening. They tried to help by doing things to cheer me up—going out to dinner, going shopping, going for a walk. Then, after their attempts failed, they became irritated with me and basically told me to "snap out of it." In fact, that's pretty much what everyone said, "Just snap out of it." Which of course made me feel even more alone and depressed. And I realize now—after years of therapy—that telling someone with clinical depression to snap out of it is akin to blaming the person for his or her illness. So not only did I have an emotional illness, but I was being blamed for it as well. It's pretty ironic; I can laugh about the lunacy of it now.

And then one day I started feeling better. I don't know why or if anything spurred it. But I began to be able to enjoy some things again. I was able to laugh now and then instead of wanting to cry all day. And that's what I later learned: that depressions will often naturally resolve on their own after three to six months. I began to get my energy back, and getting out of bed in the morning was no longer a chore. I felt motivated to go back to school for a higher degree. And I did and was pretty successful in most of my endeavors for the next five years. I got my master's degree in education and began teaching in a local elementary school. I married the man I had been dating for two years, and we had a wonderful baby boy.

Everything in my life was going really well—better than well—until I started feeling sick again. And I slid into the same kind of depression I had experienced five years earlier. Only this time, my husband urged me to see a doctor, who put me on medication just when the new class of antidepressants—the SSRIs (selective serotonin reuptake inhibitors)—had come out. And about a month after starting the medication, I began feeling better. After yet another month, I was feeling like myself again.

I've experienced two more depressive episodes since then, each lasting about three to four months. And by this time, I'm much better prepared to deal with them. I know that I have chronic episodic depression and that it's likely that I'll experience more than one recurrence in the years to come. But I know that this is the natural course of this illness and that I can endure the periods when daily life feels awful. I also know that these periods will lift in time and that I'll feel like myself again.

This illness has probably made me a more compassionate person than I otherwise would have been. Because now I understand what others go through when they suffer—I understand it first hand. I think that I'm much more patient with people and with my kids at school because I can empathize with their difficulties. I see other teachers losing patience or becoming irritated with kids who are having difficulty either academically or personally. But it's very easy for me to put myself in those kids' shoes. And my heart just goes out to them. It's almost as if I can feel the pain they're feeling. And I think I can do this because of what I've been through with my own depressions. When I feel someone else's pain, my first urge is to help them—to try to stop the pain. And if I can't do that, then at least I can let them know that I understand and I care. I wish that I never had to experience the depressions I've gone through. But I also realize that, if I didn't go through them, I wouldn't be who I am today. And I wouldn't have this ability to step into someone else's shoes and feel their pain.

Learning to have compassion for myself was much harder and took longer—and it's still an ongoing process. Ten years ago I wasn't very compassionate with myself. I held myself to perfectionistic, rigid standards that were almost impossible for me to live up to. And consequently, I felt like a failure much of the time, even though to others it must have looked like I was achieving a lot. I think that one of the most important things for me to learn was to let go of perceived failures and stop beating myself up for not being perfect.

I also learned that I truly deserved to treat myself with compassion and that it was my responsibility to behave in a loving way toward myself. For most of my life, I never felt deserving of compassion. I don't know why. I guess I still felt that something was wrong with me because of my depression. Maybe I thought that I was damaged and that I had created problems for my family because of my illness—that I had made them suffer because of me. I realized that I had to let that go and stop beating myself up for my illness. I learned to do this by training myself to become aware of the negative thoughts that run through my brain, thoughts like "You're no good. You're just a problem for others. You can't do anything right." I had a bag full of these thoughts—they seemed never ending when I first began to become consciously aware of them. And I learned to challenge these negative thoughts: "I am a good person. I do many things competently."

It took several years and a great deal of patience and persistence to come to the point where I could stop my negative thoughts before they started running away from me and then challenge them with a positive thought that's reality based. But it's still an everyday practice.

I've also stopped blaming myself for my illness and the way it's affected my family. It's an unfortunate part of my genetic makeup, but it certainly isn't something that I caused or can control beyond taking my medication. So I've forgiven myself for not being the perfect mom or wife or daughter. Because I realize that I try my best to carry out my responsibilities—I do the best I can. No one's perfect. Forgiving myself for my illness also has enabled me to forgive others who may have inadvertently hurt me because they didn't understand what depression is like—all the people who told me that I should snap out it, that I should smile, or that I was just seeking attention. I understand now that they said these things out of ignorance, out of having little or no understanding of what it's like to go through a depression. I've let go of my anger for these incidents as well. Because I understand now that these people didn't mean to hurt me; they didn't know how to help in a more appropriate way and probably couldn't deal with their own feelings of helplessness concerning my illness.

And when I started forgiving myself, and then others, so many things seemed OK that used to bother me. It was a release to let go of the blame that I always carried around. And I found that when I released this blame, I had even more compassion for others. Because then I realized that people act hurtful only when they feel helpless and unlovable. As long as I stayed in a place where I felt deserving of compassion, and I could remember to treat myself with gentleness and kindness, then I could survive. And when I have trouble remembering this, then I seek help from someone who understands how a depression can color your perspective in a very negative way.

Exercise 1: Exploring Our Ideas About Compassion

Many of us have difficulty treating ourselves with compassion. Such a skill is not one we were likely to learn in school or from our parents or religious figures. In fact, many of us have difficulty believing that we truly deserve to treat ourselves with compassion. In our society, men often experience greater difficulty treating themselves compassionately, because compassion is often thought of as a feminine quality that negates strength and stoicism. It is important, then, to first explore your ideas about compassion. Ask yourself these questions, and then explore your answers in your journal:

 As a child, what were you taught about the idea of compassion? Many religions teach the importance of compassion for others, but the idea of treating oneself with compassion is commonly alien. Is this true for you? Did your parents treat themselves and each other compassionately? Did their parents?

 What would it mean to treat yourself compassionately? The idea of compassion implies that we learn to be gentle with ourselves and with our efforts to make life meaningful and livable and that we act in loving ways toward ourselves. It also implies that we learn to be gentle with and forgiving of our perceived weaknesses, mistakes, or failures. Treating ourselves compassionately does not mean that we engage in self-indulgence or behave with a me-first attitude. It does not mean that we seek to meet our needs at the expense of others. Rather, treating ourselves compassionately means that we learn to care for ourselves in ways that nurture our spirit, mind, and body. Again, the idea of nurturing is commonly equated with feminine qualities, and men may have greater difficulty learning to nurture themselves. It is important to understand whether you value the concept of self-compassion, or whether you were raised to be hard on yourself—to drive yourself to reach unrealistic, perfectionistic standards.

🌿 If you have difficulty with the idea of treating yourself compassionately, think of the compassion you hold for those who are most dear to you. Can you imagine extending that same compassion to yourself? Has there been anyone in your life who treated you with compassion? If so, who was this person, and how did he or she demonstrate compassion in everyday acts? Can you extend the compassion that person held for you to yourself? Can you treat yourself in the same compassionate ways he or she treated you?

If you have not had the experience of knowing someone who treated you compassionately, imagine that a coach, mentor, or teacher has entered your life—someone who accepts and loves you completely. Imagine how this person would treat you. What would he or she say? How would he or she act? Explore the answers to these questions in your writing. Imagine that this mentor is teaching you how to act toward yourself in loving ways. How would this mentor teach you to behave toward yourself each day?

Now imagine that this mentor will accompany you every day for the next year to help you learn self-compassion. Let him or her become the voice in your mind that challenges you when you treat yourself in harsh, unloving ways and that urges you to remember to take the time you need to care for yourself—to nurture your spirit, mind, and body. Each day in your journal record the ways you were compassionate with yourself. It also may be helpful to work with a therapist or trusted confidant who can help challenge you to learn self-compassion.

Use mindfulness training to catch yourself when you are acting in unloving ways toward yourself. Counteract each unloving act or thought with ones that show self-compassion. Practice this until you become adept at replacing unloving acts with self-kindness.

Stop periodically during your day to ask yourself, "Am I treating myself with compassion right now? How can I change my behaviors or thoughts to be more self-compassionate?"

Exercise 2: Identifying Ways to Treat Ourselves With Compassion

Too often, self-compassion can become an abstract concept with no direct relevance to our daily lives. In Exercise 1, you identified what compassion would look and feel like if it were demonstrated by another person. Now, generate a list of behaviors and thought processes through which you can practice self-kindness. Your list may address specific behaviors, such as "Taking better care of my body through exercise, eating right, and getting enough sleep" or "Nurturing my mind by reading more." Your list also may address specific thought processes, such as "Not berating myself when I have made a mistake" or "Not blaming myself for being sick." Then, do the following:

🖎 Identify specific ways that you can be compassionate with yourself. Think of behaviors and thoughts that will enable you to nurture your spirit, mind, and body, and list these in your journal.

🖎 Try to choose one specific behavior to put into practice each week. Record how you feel before and after engaging in that behavior.

Exercise 3: Practicing Greater Compassion With Others

Once we have learned to be compassionate with ourselves, extending that compassion to others becomes easier. People often find that greater compassion for others enhances all of their relationships, including intimate relationships, work relationships, friendships, and relationships with neighbors. It is easy to be compassionate with those we love; however, having compassion for those we are in conflict with is more challenging. When others treat us in disparaging or disrespectful ways, our first response is often anger. By becoming angry, we frequently carry the conflict further. What if we could learn to step back and understand that the other person feels violated, disrespected, or unheard? And what if we remembered that the needs of that other person are no more or less important than our own?

When you are in conflict with another, step back and remember that the individual likely feels disrespected or unheard. Instead of responding in anger, tell the person in a nonattacking manner that you realize that he or she feels that his or her needs have not been met and that you are trying to understand how he or she feels. If that person attacks you, refrain from attacking back. Instead, ask for clarification of how that person feels and what he or she wants. Ask yourself if there is a way to resolve the conflict that honors the needs of all involved.

The Buddhists practice several techniques to enhance compassion for others. (See "Further Reading" for resources on Buddhism.) One involves imagining a person for whom we already have great compassion. In Buddhist tradition it is common to hold great compassion for one's mother, who made sacrifices so that one's life could be enhanced. Once Buddhist practitioners have a mental image of the mother and can feel compassion for her, they then practice extending those same feelings of compassion to other individuals, particularly ones who are not as easy to find likable. Think of a person for whom you hold great compassion. When you can fully feel your compassion for this person, try to extend that compassion to someone else. First, begin with someone you feel affection toward. When you can feel the compassion strongly, try to transfer these feelings to others you are in conflict with.

Exercise 4: Learning to Be More Forgiving of Ourselves

One of the things our society practices backward is forgiveness. We often believe that we can forgive others when we have not yet learned to forgive ourselves. The ability to forgive others is dependent on our ability to forgive ourselves first. Ask yourself the following questions, and explore your answers in your journal:

💘 Are you hypercritical of yourself and your behaviors? Do you have difficulty forgiving yourself for mistakes or missed opportunities?

💘 Do you feel guilty for being ill? Or do you fear that you are letting others down because of your illness? Do you feel guilty because you can no longer take responsibility and care for your loved ones in ways that you were once accustomed to?

℘ Identify the qualities in yourself and in your life about which you are most unforgiving. Where did you learn to hold yourself to such standards? Think back to the behaviors of your parents (and their parents), schoolteachers, religious figures, siblings, and peers. Can you remember instances in which any of these people stated, "I'll never forgive myself for . . ."? Or "I'll never forgive so-and-so for . . ."? When did these instances occur? And how did they affect the way you learned to view forgiveness?

Learning to make peace with ourselves first requires the acknowledgment that we are all fallible beings who make mistakes as part of the natural course of life. It requires that we view mistakes and lost opportunities as part of the personal learning and growth process. The following steps are useful for making peace with ourselves:

℘ Identify the mistakes and lost opportunities in your life that you have difficulty forgiving yourself for. Identify any other events that you hold yourself responsible for in an unforgiving way. It is helpful to list these in your journal.

℘ Go through your list and, one by one, try to reconsider how you feel about each experience. Try to reframe the experience as the consequence of not being adequately prepared to handle that situation or not having enough knowledge or understanding to make better choices at the time. Instead of blaming yourself, try to understand that you did the best you could given the resources and level of knowledge that you had.

℘ Acknowledge that you are not bad for having made the decisions you did at the time. Recognize that, today, you would make different choices based on the greater level of understanding you now have.

❧ Practice mindfulness training by catching yourself whenever you have negative thoughts about self-forgiveness. Learn to catch thoughts in which you reproach yourself for some perceived mistake or problem. Practice replacing such thoughts with ones in which you acknowledge that everyone makes mistakes, that mistakes are a natural part of learning, and that you are doing the best you can given the resources and understanding you have.

❧ Learn to catch thoughts in which you blame yourself for being unable to meet some rigid standard. Acknowledge that you do not have to be perfect—no one is or ever will be. When challenging unrealistically high standards, it is often helpful to first list them. Identify the specific standards you hold that may be unrealistically high and stringent. Next to each standard, describe a modified version that is more realistic and reasonable for you to meet. When you catch thoughts in which you attempt to impose your old, unrealistic standards on yourself, replace the old standards with your revised versions.

It is often helpful to work with a therapist when attempting to modify unrealistic standards. We commonly require help in identifying standards that are unrealistic, because they may operate in our lives unconsciously. A skilled therapist can help us understand how unrealistic standards maintain our self-berating behaviors and can also help us learn to replace such standards with more reasonable ones.

Exercise 5: Making Peace With Others

People who transform their lives through illness or disability commonly find that healing is impeded by holding on to grudges and past grievances. Forgiving others appears to be a necessary ingredient for emotional healing, and there is some evidence for physical healing as well. (See "Further Reading" for resources on healing through forgiveness.) Once we learn how to forgive ourselves, it is easier to extend that same forgiveness to others. Ask yourself these questions:

🖋 Are you the type of person who holds grudges and has difficulty forgiving?

🖋 Are there people in your life with whom you have severed connection because of a past grievance?

🖋 Are there people with whom you are presently in conflict?

You must first decide if you are willing to forgive those with whom you are in conflict. Forgiving others does not necessarily mean that you also will mend broken relationships. Forgiveness requires only that you no longer feel resentment and anger toward those people and the events that created the conflict between you. Thus, you can forgive others, even if they do not forgive you. The key to forgiveness is to empty your heart of bitterness and to fill it with compassion.

You must decide if you wish to mend severed relationships. Many people in the process of transforming their lives through illness do not feel completely settled until they heal bonds with people whom they still hold dear. Consider doing the following:

🖋 Make a list of the severed relationships and conflicts you have experienced in your life.

🖋 Determine if you are still holding on to resentment and anger over these situations. If so, do you wish to release your resentment and anger in the forgiveness process?

🖋 Think back to each experience you listed, one at a time. Can you acknowledge that the person with whom you experienced conflict did not understand how to act more compassionately toward you at the time? Try to remember how you felt about that person before the conflict occurred.

Try to recall the feelings of friendship and love that you shared. Stay focused on those feelings rather than on the anger that came later.

Remember, people make mistakes and act in hurtful ways because they do not understand the consequences for all involved. And remember that forgiving does not mean condoning hurtful behavior. Rather, it allows us to release our bitterness over what occurred.

Sometimes it helps to imagine having a conversation with that person in which you share your feelings about what happened and express your forgiveness. It also can be helpful to have this conversation with a therapist who can role-play the person with whom you have severed connection. This type of therapeutic technique can be particularly helpful when you are trying to forgive others who are no longer alive. Writing down this conversation in a journal also can be cathartic.

FOUR

ACCEPTING LIFE AS IT UNFOLDS AND LETTING GO OF EXPECTATIONS

The people who transformed their lives through illness or disability commonly spoke of the need to accept life as it unfolds—to accept their illness or disability, to accept the course that their lives have taken. To accept life as it unfolds, they had to learn to relinquish their attachment to specific expectations. Illness brings with it the understanding that nothing in life can be predicted but change, and those who can find meaning in life despite illness or disability can best live with uncertainty. When the people interviewed for this book released their attachment to specific outcomes and expectations, they also released their struggle and conflict with perceived adversity. They stopped resisting their experience and instead looked deeper into what opportunities their experience brought them. They also ended their attempts to control every detail of their lives and became less preoccupied with the minutiae of life.

When these individuals began to accept their life as it unfolded, instead of resisting it, they found that they were able to accept what came with greater equanimity. They learned to live life at the ocean's edge, developing greater confidence in their ability to get back up if a wave knocked them down. They realized that they could more easily ride out the waves of a storm, even knowing that a greater storm would likely follow. Some said that they lost their fear of the unknown and, with it, their need to control it. Others observed that, when they released their attachment to specific expectations, they also released their need to control others, allowing them greater opportunity to enjoy just being with their loved ones without expectations.

Bob's Acceptance of Life as It Unfolded

In 1989, when Bob was 39, he sustained a spinal cord injury in an automobile accident when his car was pushed off the road by a truck driver who had fallen asleep at the wheel. Bob was on a business trip, and it was in the early morning hours when a tractor-trailer pulled close behind him and thrust his car through a steel barrier and down a steep embankment. As a result of the accident, Bob was paralyzed from the waist down. He spent four months in the hospital regaining his strength and learning to perform basic activities of daily living without the use of his legs.

ALL MY LIFE I'VE BEEN A WORRIER. So it was no irony that I went into the insurance business after college. And being in insurance, I saw all kinds of traumas that can happen to people—all kinds of freak accidents and acts of nature. And I guess that made me worry even more. I worried about the future. I worried about my kids and how they'd turn out. I worried about the economy and if I'd earn enough to provide my family with a good life. I worried about my job and if I could lose it. And I tried to plan everything. I thought if I had everything planned out, I could prevent the things I worried about.

But even after being in the insurance business and seeing all of the bad things that can happen to people, and despite all of my worries, I still never thought that something like this would happen to me. Despite all my worries and all my planning to avert my worries, I just wasn't prepared for my injury. When it first happened, I really thought that my life was over. I just couldn't see how I could live like this. It just wasn't in my plans for a happy life. And I was very angry for a long time, because all of a sudden my life took a turn that I didn't expect or want. That was the hardest thing: reckoning what happened with the expectations I had for my life. Learning to use a wheelchair and putting on my pants without standing up didn't turn out to be the toughest part of all this. The really hard part was learning to accept what happened and move on with my life. And to give up my attachment to the way I thought life would be.

In the first months after the accident, the thought of not being able to walk was overwhelming to me. Not being able to play football with my son or walk my daughter down the aisle when she'd marry. Not being able to have sex with my wife. Not being able to get up from a chair on my own and walk across the room. I simply couldn't imagine that my life could ever be happy again. I was very attached to my body and to being able to play sports and finish the renovations I was making on the house. I was used to meeting people and looking them in the eye straight on, not sitting three feet below them in a wheelchair. When I first went back to work, shaking hands with someone while they were standing and I was sitting made me uncomfortable and ashamed. I had a tremendously hard time accepting what had happened to me and that my life was not going to turn out as I had planned.

My wife and I—our whole lives had to change. We had to move to a ranch house so I wouldn't have to deal with stairs. We renovated the bathrooms and kitchen so that the countertops were lower so I could reach them. I had to learn how to drive a car with hand controls instead of a brake pedal. My office at work had to be redesigned to accommodate a wheelchair. And with every change, I had to give up my desire that things remain the way they always were.

But after several years of living with a spinal cord injury, and with the considerable help of my dear wife and some excellent rehab therapists, I realized that I could have the life I wanted; it was just going to look a little different from what I expected. Most of the things I wanted I could still have, but in a different way. I could play wheelchair sports with my son; in fact, for six years I played on a wheelchair basketball team. I escorted my daughter down the aisle in my wheelchair when she got married. Sex with my wife is not the same, but I learned that sex doesn't have to be just intercourse. I still have my workshop; it's an adapted workshop so that all of my power tools are at the level of my wheelchair. And for the past several years I've built custom furniture.

Most of the expectations I had for myself came to pass—they just look a little different from what I imagined. And that's been the toughest thing I had to learn: that the more I couldn't let go of my expectations, the more struggle and disappointment I experienced when life didn't turn out exactly as planned. Instead, when I'm open to the possibilities of what may happen—instead of expecting things to turn out the way I want—then life isn't a struggle as much. Don't get me wrong; it's still a struggle. But it's a little easier to accept when you don't have rigid plans.

I used to have my whole life planned out, down to the year and day I would retire and how my wife and I would spend our retirement. None of those plans involved having a spinal cord injury. When it first happened, I really resisted the idea that life could ever be livable again. Now, after 15 years of living with this type of injury—I'm 54 now—I no longer feel the need to plan the future. And I'm not as worried about the future as I used to be—maybe because I survived not only the accident but also the trauma afterward. Today, I'm much more apt to see what life brings instead of holding onto rigid expectations, because I've learned that life never brings what you expect anyway. But it often brings chances to meet your goals in ways you never expected. Life ends up looking very different from what you imagined. Still, if you can imagine it, somehow the opportunity will come for you to realize your goals—but those goals will just look a little different from what you originally imagined. And I've learned that if you can be OK with that, then life doesn't have to be a constant struggle. It's easier to let life happen, to accept it, and figure out a way to live with it—like the old proverb about flowing with the stream instead of fighting it.

When I look back, I had so many expectations for my life—expectations about how much money I should make, about what I should accomplish in my career, about how many grandchildren I wanted. Now I realize that none of those expectations really mattered or helped me prepare for what life dished out. Being able to accept life, to accept what happens, to be flexible so that you can adjust to the turns in the road that you didn't foresee up ahead—that's one of the greatest life lessons that someone can learn. And I guess that's the lesson I learned from having this injury.

Exercise 1: Identifying Our Attachment to Specific Events and Outcomes

Living with illness or disability involves living with uncertainty, and living with uncertainty evokes anxiety, fear, and an instinctive need to control our circumstances. Buddhists and Taoists suggest that one method to live with uncertainty involves learning to be more comfortable with the way in which our life unfolds—to be able to accept what comes rather than having rigid expectations for every situation and then feeling unsettled and disappointed when life does not turn out as planned. (See "Further Reading" for resources on Buddhism and Taoism.) Record the following in your journal:

🍂 Identify your attachment to specific events, circumstances, and relationships. Identify the expectations that you have for these events and relationships. Are your expectations so rigid that you have difficulty tolerating instances when they are not met or when others have different expectations that conflict with your own?

🍂 Consider how you learned to react to unfulfilled expectations. How did your parents (or those who raised you) react to their own unmet expectations? Were they accepting of how life unfolded, or did they resist it? When you were a child and you expressed disappointment in response to unmet expectations, were those feelings encouraged or discouraged?

🍂 As an adult, how have you typically dealt with your own unfulfilled expectations? If you resist undesired life circumstances, ask yourself if this has caused greater difficulty in your life than if you were able to be more accepting.

🍂 Consider how your life might feel if your expectations (for events in the present and future) remain unfulfilled. Often, we believe that our lives will be unbearable and unlivable if our expectations are not satisfied, but then we find that life is indeed still livable, despite our initial fears for the worst. We may have felt similarly before our illness—perhaps we believed that we could never live with illness. But after illness enters our lives, we discover that we can indeed continue to live and find meaning in everyday life. Next to each expectation you identified above, list the fears you have—for your life and for your loved ones' lives—if those expectations were to go unmet. What might be the worst-case scenario?

 Considering the expectations you have identified, try to imagine what you might learn if those expectations remained unsatisfied. We are often challenged to learn and grow through events we perceive as adversity. Think of the positive ways in which you may be challenged to change if the expectations that you identified do not materialize. List positive outcomes for all of your unsatisfied expectations; record these next to your list of worst-case scenarios so that you can begin to compare the two perspectives—what you fear most versus how you may grow if it comes to pass.

Exercise 2: Practicing Accepting Our Experience as It Unfolds

How can one practice accepting one's experience as it unfolds? After loosening our grip on rigid expectations, the next step involves reassessing the opportunities that past adversity has brought to us and disciplining our minds to consider possible learning opportunities in the face of seeming tribulation. We may initially react to hardship with disappointment, anger, and sadness. But to truly learn to accept life as it unfolds, we must develop the habit of considering the unexpected opportunities each adverse situation may hold for us that we may never have experienced otherwise. We may not be able to understand how adversity has brought positive opportunity into our lives until months or even years later, when we are better able to assess the situation in its entirety (and when we have secured a greater emotional distance).

The ongoing practice of considering positive opportunity in the face of challenge offers two benefits. First, with consistent practice, it allows us to more readily identify and understand the learning opportunities that are presented to us. Second, as our belief strengthens that positive outcome will result from hardship, we will be better able to survive adversity and take advantage of its opportunities. In your journal, compile a list of the disappointments you have experienced in the past five years. Next to each item, write down the unexpected opportunities for growth that have emerged in each situation. Consider the opportunities for growth that appeared during your illness.

When you observe this list as a whole, can you identify repeated learning opportunities that presented themselves through different life situations? In other words, can we learn the same lessons from different life circumstances? Because change often requires a lengthy period of time, we frequently benefit from multiple challenging experiences that collectively help us experience growth-promoting change.

Exercise 3: Releasing Our Need for Control Over the Moment and Others

Another method to practice greater acceptance of life as it unfolds involves learning to release our control over the moment and over others in our immediate environment. Many of us are natural planners and feel more secure when we have orchestrated a situation to gain greater control over it. Others have dispositions that allow them to be more spontaneous and flexible; their need to mold situations to their desires is not as great. Examine to what degree you feel that you need to exert control over specific events and over other people in your life. Is it difficult for you to be flexible and to go with the flow?

The Buddhists speak of exercising greater fluidity in one's actions and behaviors—in other words, flowing around impediments instead of fighting against them and creating resistance and conflict. (See "Further Reading" for resources on Buddhism.) Practice being with others without expectation. To do this you must first become aware of the expectations you hold for others. Identify a specific situation that is occurring presently in your life and determine who is involved. What expectations do you have of the people in this situation? What expectations do you have of yourself? When you write them down in your journal, do these expectations seem reasonable and realistic? Or are these expectations unrealistic? Are you expecting people to demonstrate behaviors and skills that are beyond their capacity (as demonstrated by their behavior in past situations)? If so, you must recognize that you have created conditions that are likely to bring disappointment.

Imagine holding no specific expectations for particular events and others. To begin to practice this skill, choose one event that will occur in the upcoming week. It should be an event that does not evoke strong emotions. In your mind, envision yourself participating in the event as it unfolds. Practice imagining that you do not hold any specific expectations concerning how the situation will turn out. When it is time for the event to actually occur, try to participate in it without expectation. Do not berate yourself if you experience difficulty practicing this skill on initial attempts. Just continue to practice with events about which you do not feel strongly. When you can successfully participate in an event without expectation, proceed to events that evoke stronger emotions.

Exercise 4: Relinquishing Inappropriate Control and Responsibility

Throughout life, we find ourselves in situations in which we have inappropriately assumed control and responsibility for events and others. Perhaps we were the most competent person to handle a specific situation. Or others may have handed their responsibility over to us because of our competence and willingness to assume control. Over time, inappropriate control and responsibility—particularly when other adults should be sharing in the collective responsibility—become burdensome, and we do not know how to end the cycle of our own participation. (The concept of inappropriate responsibility does not involve one's responsibility for children, which is entirely appropriate; this concept applies to adults who have assumed excessive responsibility for other adults.)

We may feel guilty about relinquishing control and responsibility. We may fear that situations will unravel without our vigilance and direction. Or we may feel that it is unfair to relinquish responsibility to others who have become dependent on us. Such dependence, however, does not promote growth either in others or in ourselves—over-dependence prevents individuals from growing and developing their own independence and resourcefulness. We may also find satisfaction in having others remain dependent on us; such feelings may allow us to feel appreciated and valued. Ultimately, however, others' dependence causes us to feel burdened and angry, and that anger often emerges in unconscious ways that cause conflict for all involved.

Relinquishing inappropriate control and responsibility is necessary for our acceptance of life as it unfolds in accordance with its own natural course—without our manipulation. The

Buddhist practice of nonaction involves the belief that the more we try to control a situation, the more it escapes our control. (See "Further Reading" for resources on Buddhism.) The more we attempt to manipulate events and people according to our own desires, the more situations will turn out in ways opposite from what we initially desired. To relinquish inappropriate control and responsibility, it is necessary to become more comfortable with the practice of nonaction. These activities may be beneficial:

❦ First, identify the people in your life for whom you have taken inappropriate control and responsibility.

❦ Practice releasing your need to control the person or his or her actions in a specific situation. Identify one event for which you have assumed inappropriate control and responsibility. (Choose a situation involving other adults rather than children for whom you are responsible.) Begin with an event whose outcome is not critical. Instead of managing the people involved in the situation as you normally would—by exerting control, directing events, and fixing problems—allow events to unfold without your intervention. Did you find that you could participate in this situation and repress your need to exert your own will over what transpired? Did you find yourself making rationalizations for your need to exert your influence over others? For example, "Things would not have turned out well if I did not intervene," "The situation would have gotten out of control if I did not act," or "Others are depending on me to help—I can't let them down." Did you find yourself taking responsibility for a collective situation in which the participation of others determines the outcome for everyone (including yourself)? Or did you find that the situation worked out despite your fears?

✒ When you can participate in specific situations whose outcomes are not critical without exerting your need to control others, then proceed to situations whose outcomes are more serious. Choose situations for which you have characteristically taken greater responsibility than other (adult) participants who should be sharing equal responsibility and who may have become dependent on your willingness to assume control. To relinquish our need to control others, we must first give back responsibility to them.

Exercise 5: Rejecting the Idea That We Have to Fix Ourselves or Others

Accepting life also means rejecting the idea that we and others need to be fixed. Western culture promotes the idea that people are broken and need help fixing the problems in their lives and in their psyches. Viewing our lives from a perspective of inadequacy and deficit promotes the perception that we are broken and unacceptable. This perception naturally extends to others whom we also find to be lacking.

We may feel particularly broken if we are ill, as our society instills the belief that illness and wholeness are antithetical. Our search for a cure may in part underlie an effort to restore a sense of wholeness to our lives. The ability to feel whole, however, depends more on our ability to accept ourselves and the course that our lives have taken, in spite of the presence of illness.

To accept life as it has unfolded, we must cultivate the practice of viewing our lives from a perspective of acceptance, adequacy, and wholeness rather than inadequacy and deficit. It is first necessary to become aware of deficit thinking, which is characterized by the belief that one's life is inadequate and lacking and that one is unacceptable. These activities may be helpful:

🍃 In your journal, list the aspects of your life about which you feel a sense of inadequacy (in other words, aspects that you believe require correction).

🍃 Now, try to change your perspective from inadequacy to acceptability. Next to each condition of lacking that you identified, describe how this condition contributes positively to the wholeness of your life. For example, if you are ill and have identified illness as a condition of lacking, you may instead view your illness as an opportunity to become closer to family members and to learn to accept help from others. The goal is to modify your thinking style from a continuous finding of fault to acceptance that the conditions of your life contribute to the greater good of your life as a whole.

When we can begin to accept that our life circumstances, no matter how seemingly negative, have benefited our life's journey, we can begin to extend that acceptance to other people. We no longer view others as broken or feel compelled to fix them. We accept that the qualities about a person that we find difficult to accept are our own problem. If a relationship has not been emotionally healthy, rather than attempting to change that person, we either accept those qualities or remove ourselves from interaction. We also do not allow others to attempt to fix what they perceive as broken in us.

🍃 Identify another whom you have, in the past, attempted to fix. Describe the qualities of that person that you perceived as inadequate or lacking. Now, try to view these qualities from the opposite perspective, from one of wholeness and acceptability. How did these qualities—which you found to be unacceptable—contribute positively to that person's life? For example, if you find your spouse to be irritatingly tenacious, can you also perceive how this persistence enabled other accomplishments (such as material comfort)?

Over time, you can use mindfulness training to catch and counteract deficit thinking. Recording this process in your journal helps facilitate the practice and mastery of these skills.

FIVE

LEARNING TO BE
PRESENT IN AND
APPRECIATE THE MOMENT

The people who found greater meaning in their lives through the experience of illness or disability said that one of the most important keys to greater daily life satisfaction amidst pain involves finding meaning in the very moment they are living—not tomorrow or next week. Being present in and appreciating the moment requires the ability to focus fully on what is happening now; it requires that one stop projecting oneself into the past and regretting or longing for it. It also requires that one stop projecting oneself into the future and worrying about it.

Instead, these people, who had learned to be fully in and to appreciate the present, said that they live each moment as it comes, out of an awareness that the only real importance lies in the present, for our greatest opportunity to make life-affirming changes lies in the present moment. Those who focused on the present moment and appreciated its opportunities were more able to appreciate the ordinary everyday events that make life meaningful. These people grounded themselves in the small joys of life. They learned to celebrate the relationships and gifts in their lives in the present instead of focusing on what was not there. Because they had experienced being stripped to the essentials of human life, their values became clearer, and the satisfactions of a loved one's touch or the presence of a beloved pet in the present moment became more important than worrying about something that may or may not occur in the future.

Joan's Experience of Learning to Live in the Present Moment

Two months after Joan's 47th birthday, she learned that she had non-Hodgkin's lymphoma—a disease involving malignancy of the lymphatic system. Like many people who receive a diagnosis of cancer, Joan was frightened, despite her doctor's reassurances that the cancer had been caught early and that her prognosis was good.

WHEN I RECEIVED MY DIAGNOSIS—non-Hodgkin's lymphoma—I didn't even know what it was. It sounded like something horrific, and of course when I heard "cancer," I think I became so terrified that I just stopped listening further to anything my doctor was saying. I think that for quite a long time I was captured by my fear. I'd wake up in the morning in a panic. Or in the middle of the night, I'd awake from nightmares in a cold sweat. I teach high school English, and I'd be in class and a wave of anxiety would come over me, and all I wanted to do was get out of that classroom. I couldn't concentrate. My lectures were sparse and disorganized. Grading high school English papers is not exactly smooth reading, so you can imagine the time I had concentrating on my students' papers once I found out that I had cancer.

When I started my treatment, I didn't feel any better. In fact, for a while I felt worse. The medication had awful side effects on my stomach, and the radiation made me nauseous and tired. For a while I couldn't keep food in at either end. So I was convinced that I was dying. And I became very depressed, just very despondent, even though my doctors told me that my prognosis was good. Cancer runs in my mother's line, and I started thinking that I had inherited the genes for cancer and that, even if the non-Hodgkin's lymphoma was cured, I'd experience another form of cancer. My life had become overwhelming for me. I was seeing my primary care doctor, the oncologist, and the psychiatrist—I had at least two doctor's appointments every week for a while. I was feeling pretty sick physically and mentally. And I just couldn't live like this.

At some point I think I said to myself, "Look, you can either live with this fear and with this sickness, or your life can be over and you can forget about enjoying anything ever again." I'm not sure exactly how I got to the point where I said, "I can accept this. I can make the most of my life while living with this pain, whatever happens." I realized that my life had become so overwhelming that I had to stop the way I was going and start dealing with one thing at a time—because that's all I could handle. And I realized that I had to start living my life in the present moment instead of worrying about the future and how sick I might get. Or whether the cancer would return or spread to some other part of my body. I started thinking that if I didn't make the most of now, I'd have nothing, because I wasn't all that sure what my future would be like. And I realized that I at least had my life right now in the present, that I had to start enjoying the things that were OK in my day, like playing with my dog and seeing his joy in being alive, talking on the phone with my sister, taking a walk in the sun, and just appreciating the way the sunlight streams through the tree leaves.

What my illness did for me was to stop me in my tracks and make me re-evaluate my life. It made me realize that I won't be here forever, and it forced me to start appreciating today. Really, all we have is the present moment. My illness made me understand the importance of living in the now rather than obsessing about the future. I realized that I don't want to live worrying about what awful thing might happen to me next. Right now, in this very moment, I'm OK. I can live with what's happening right now.

And that was a turning point for me—when I began to understand that if I focused on what's going on right now, I could manage. I wasn't overwhelmed because I wasn't playing out some disturbing fantasy about the future in my head. All the time I was worrying about my future, I missed out on appreciating my life in the present. And I didn't want to continue missing out on my life in the present. Life goes by too fast to miss it and to waste it by living in the future. And living that way—always worrying about the future or being upset about the past—is draining. I was draining my energy by spending most of my time worrying.

So I try not to spend my thoughts on the past or on the future anymore. Often during the day I'll have thoughts about the future—a lot of it is still about my illness. I have a doctor's appointment on the 21st of the month, and that's been coming into my mind. I find myself worrying if the cancer will return; I've been in remission for a year now. So when worries come into my mind during the day, I acknowledge them and try to bring my focus back to the present moment—what's happening right now. I try to remember that I feel OK right now, that there's no reason to get anxious. And I monitor my breathing. Often, when I feel anxious, I start breathing short, shallow breaths. So I make an effort to breathe deeply and slowly, and this helps to calm my fears and stops the roller coaster ride of my anxieties.

If you're living in the moment and concentrating on the activity before you, you're not focusing on your worries. And if you can find a sense of peace in your daily activities—folding fresh laundry that smells and feels good, eating pancakes on a Sunday morning while reading the paper—then you can feel OK rather than worrying about tomorrow or the day after or how sick you may become six months from now. My illness made me appreciate the common things in my day that I never thought twice about before and to better value how truly important these things are. I've become much more appreciative of very simple things, things like really enjoying eating a bagel with cream cheese or seeing the stars on a clear night. Or just appreciating nature and how beautiful the trees are, taking a walk with my dog, listening to my niece's teenage dramas. Being able to appreciate these small ordinary things—that I once didn't pay attention to—has enriched my life. And I think that's what my life is really all about. My life is a thousand of these little things that are all put together like a mosaic. And being able to experience enjoyment from each one helps me to have a better life.

I also realized that, before my illness, my life was very out of balance. I bordered on being a workaholic, and I was definitely heading down a track of doing too much instead of just being. In fact, I used to feel that I was wasting time if I wasn't doing something—grading papers, reading Shakespearean plays, cleaning out the garage. The list of things that needed to get done was endless. But now I can say to myself, "So what if the dishes don't get done right now? So what if I don't grade those papers until Wednesday?" What does it matter? It doesn't. Now when I wake up in the morning, instead of thinking, "How much can I get done today?" I think, "How can I live a balanced life today? What can I do to bring some degree of joy to my day today?" And I realize that's what it's all about—not how much I can get done. Who can remember what I did a week ago or a month ago? It doesn't even really matter. What matters is that I'm able to appreciate the moment before me and to find peace and comfort in the common, ordinary, familiar things that make up my life.

Exercise 1: Waking up in the Present Moment

Many of us tend to sleep through our present moments—to experience life unconsciously until some crisis evokes pain or distress. We press on through our days either by rote or in a crisis mode. How many of us truly experience each moment consciously? How often do we find that a car ride or a conversation has transpired without our full attention? We recognize only later that we missed fully experiencing such moments because our thoughts were elsewhere. Waking up in the present moment involves becoming conscious of immediate events—and our feelings in response to those events—as we experience them. To be present in and appreciate the moment, we must learn to bring our focus to each event before us.

One exercise to increase our consciousness in the present moment involves becoming aware of all of our sensations as we are experiencing them. Stop what you are doing right now and observe your sensations. Consciously note what you are seeing, hearing, tasting, smelling, and touching. The next time you are involved in any mundane activity—whether it be driving to work, getting dressed, or preparing a meal—consciously observe each of your sensations. Try to become more fully aware of ordinary events that you typically overlook or ignore, such as the feel of a comb as it weaves through your hair or the smell of clean clothing as you dress. Practice becoming conscious of all of your sensations at least once a day. Gradually you will learn to experience your sensations at a more conscious level, and this will heighten your ability to fully experience the present moment.

This practice can be especially important when we are experiencing physical pain as a result of illness. Often the experience of pain can dominate our perception and inhibit our ability to remain conscious of other sensations. The ability to heighten our focus on sensations other than pain can sometimes help us manage pain. If you are experiencing physical pain, try to spend one period per day focusing on nonpainful sensations. For example, while you brush your teeth, become consciously aware of how the toothpaste tastes on your tongue. Observe its scent and attend to the feel and sound of the bristles as they rub against your teeth. Notice the whiteness of the paste as it liquefies in your mouth. With continued practice, you can become more adept at using this activity to consciously decrease your focus on pain.

Another exercise that can increase our focus on the present moment is to practice focusing on the sensation of breathing. We often do not realize how constricted and shallow our breathing has become. Shallow, short breaths are particularly common under conditions of stress, pain, and anxiety about the future. One Buddhist practice of breath control involves the following steps: Inhale deeply as you count slowly to five. Feel the sensation of your chest and stomach expanding and rising. Pause before exhalation. Exhale slowly for a count of five. Observe the sensation in your chest and stomach as the air is expelled. Pause again before inhalation. Repeat these steps for 10 to 15 minutes or as long as you can tolerate. Focused attention on breathing not only allows us to stay centered in the present moment but also facilitates relaxation and stress reduction. (See "Further Reading" for resources on Buddhism.)

Feeling our sensations is different from analyzing them. Sometimes we confuse the two, and we analyze our experience rather than feel it. Feeling our sensations involves being aware of our physical responses to the environment. Analyzing our experience is a cognitive phenomenon involving assessment and judgment. Often, when we are analyzing our experience—assessing and judging it—we disengage from our ability to feel the present moment. The expectations we hold about the present moment interfere with our ability to simply feel it. To enhance our awareness of the present moment, it is important to learn to separate feeling from analysis. Be certain that when you practice heightening your awareness of sensation, you do not judge those sensations.

A third exercise that encourages our conscious experience of the present moment is the Buddhist practice of eating meals in silence. (See "Further Reading" for resources on Buddhism.) We often eat meals in the midst of a variety of distractions—the television; conversation with others; or our own preoccupation, worry, and stress. In our hurried society, meals are frequently a secondary activity that we carry out while engaging in other pursuits that occupy our consciousness. Consider the circumstances in which you eat your daily meals. Do you eat meals while carrying out other activities or watching television? Do you eat as a social activity, in which conversation with others dominates your consciousness? Commonly, we sleep while we eat, and we consume food without fully experiencing the sensation of eating.

At least once a week, eat one meal in silence, trying to remain fully conscious of the eating experience. Focus on the scent of your food, the color and texture of each bite, and the way it feels in your mouth. Try to savor each food's flavor and discriminate between the tastes of the different foods on your plate. Consciously observe the temperature of the food, how it sounds as you chew it in your mouth, and the richness of the colors. Acknowledge your gratitude for having food that is both nourishing and pleasing to your senses. Offer thanks for the sensation of fullness in your stomach upon finishing your meal.

Exercise 2: Focusing on the Present Rather Than the Past or Future

Very often we miss out on the experience of the present moment because we are immersed in thoughts about the past or future. When we stop and observe our thoughts, we frequently find that we spend an inordinate amount of time worrying about the future or regretting something that happened in the past. Sometimes we are so attached to our expectations of the future that we cannot accept the present moment because it does not resemble what we hope for. Our attachment to the past—to our life before illness—also may inhibit our ability to accept the present moment as it is. How often do we spend our thoughts longing for a past that we may not have fully appreciated at the time? We should learn to value our present moments now rather than finding later that we wish we had appreciated the past as it occurred. Too often, we search for happiness somewhere in an uncertain future, rather than now, in the present moment.

Chapter 2 described the practice of mindfulness training as a technique to help increase awareness of our thoughts in the present moment. Using mindfulness training, and recording the results in your journal, try to observe your thoughts continuously for 15 minutes each day.

☙ Catch all thoughts in which your mind drifts from the present moment to the past or the future, and record them. Do you find that particular themes or events repeatedly surface in your mind? Observe how frequently you are able to maintain your thoughts in the present moment and how much of your thoughts involve the past or future.

☙ Periodically during the day, stop and use mindfulness training to observe your thoughts. Record these in your journal. Over time, you will be able to observe whether your thoughts tend to involve specific themes or events that may reflect unresolved issues needing healing. With practice, you can learn to spend at least 15 minutes each day focusing on the present moment before you and disciplining your mind to repress concerns about the past or future for this short period of time.

Exercise 3: Finding Satisfaction in the Present Moment

When we have become more adept at disciplining our minds to stay focused in the present instead of drifting to worries about the past or future, the next step involves learning to identify happiness or satisfaction in the present rather than seeking it in the future or longing for it in the past. Identifying our experience of satisfaction in the present moment commonly involves acknowledging the seemingly insignificant events that often go unnoticed but that offer comfort and contentment—the feel of a cat's fur, the sound of a friend's voice on the phone.

Chapter 1 introduced the idea of a gratitude journal, a place to acknowledge and record those events during each day for which you are thankful. In your journal, record the small, ordinary, everyday events that contribute to a sense of satisfaction in your life each day. Major life events that significantly elevate your mood do not occur every day; rather, you will more likely identify unassuming happenings that provide a sense of contentment—occurrences that you would likely otherwise overlook. This exercise helps us acknowledge the events in our everyday lives that maintain our equanimity and strengthen our resolve to continue living despite hardship. Too often we disregard these bits of happiness in our life and instead allow perceived major crises to unsettle our emotional balance. By growing accustomed to identifying the events we are grateful for each day, we can more easily recall these gifts to steady our minds in times of crisis.

Do not neglect to identify important but seemingly uneventful occasions such as meaningful interaction with others (for instance, a friendly exchange of words with the person who delivers your mail), experiences with nature (such as the pleasure of observing geese flying south), and your experience with the physical world (for example, enjoying a shower or a subway ride). At the end of the day, peruse the list of events that brought satisfaction to your life during the day. Acknowledge that, although most items on your list may be modest, these events contributed to your greater appreciation for life—they made your life easier to live today. Acknowledge that these events are gifts, and offer thanks for their presence in your life.

Exercise 4: Accepting the Present as It Is Rather Than Judging It

Being able to find satisfaction in the present moment also depends on our ability to accept the moment without expectation or attachment to outcome. How often do we find fault with our experience because it does not meet our expectations? When we judge the moment before us and compare it to some ideal standard, we lose the ability to experience the satisfactions that can contribute to our greater emotional comfort. Once we have become skilled in remaining conscious in the present moment, we need to learn to accept each moment in its own form rather than expecting it to conform to a preconceived expectation.

Some of us grew up in an environment in which almost every event was negatively judged, even events that appeared to be acceptable. We may have internalized this style of interacting with the world so that it became our customary way of thinking and responding. Examine whether your parents and family members readily judged one another and held each other to unattainable standards. Did they find fault with and criticize their experience? Were they the type of people for whom nothing was satisfactory? If you grew up in such a background and internalized it, it is important to break that style of interaction with the world and make a conscious effort to find acceptance in each experience that you have judged critically. Practice these steps:

🖌 Using mindfulness training, catch the thoughts you have in which you make a judgment about the unacceptability of the present moment. When you experience judgmental thoughts, challenge their validity. Ask yourself if the situation is truly as negative as you initially perceived it to be.

🖌 Then challenge each thought by identifying at least one thing that is acceptable about the situation you are judging. It could be as simple as the idea that the present event—which you have judged unacceptable—will come to an end in five minutes. This exercise can enable us to end our critical thought patterns and find greater acceptance in the present moment.

The Buddhists practice mindfulness training of both thought and speech. (See "Further Reading" for resources on Buddhism.) In addition to disciplining the mind to relinquish judgmental thoughts, one makes equal effort to discipline one's speech—to remove negative, hurtful words about others and events. Practice refraining from verbalizing negative comments about yourself, others, and occurrences in the present moment. As we remove such negativity from our speech, we find that our acceptance of the present moment (and of others and ourselves) becomes easier.

Exercise 5: Learning to Live One Day at a Time

Learning to be present in and appreciate the moment is connected to the idea that life is more easily lived one day at a time. Our lifestyles have become so fast-paced and chaotic that we have forgotten how to live each day as it comes without worrying about tomorrow or regretting yesterday. We have become so future oriented—saving for down payments and mortgages, building children's college funds, planning for retirement—that we have forgotten how to make the day before us meaningful. We have learned to invest a great deal in our future; we need to learn to invest as much in the present. Too often, our present days become disposable, just one of so many other throwaway products in our society.

Illness often has a way of bringing one's focus back to the present; living with an uncertain future allows us to appreciate the day we have right now. There is a saying about crossing bridges when we come to them that reflects the idea that life can best be lived only in the present moment and the fact that, when we worry about feared events in the future, we are wasting the present.

When fear about the future becomes overwhelming, we must remember to slow down and live in the present.

Acknowledge the fearful thoughts you have, and if it would be helpful, describe this fear in your journal. Much of the time, our fears revolve around some future event rather than the present moment. When we examine the present moment, we often discover that nothing is occurring presently that would contribute to our fear. Remember that what you fear is not happening in your present moment. In fact, it may never materialize.

Over the next days, when you feel overwhelmed or fearful, use the exercises in this chapter to bring your focus back to the present moment. Recognize that there is nothing happening right now to feel anxious about. Record each experience of anxiety and fear in your journal. Next to each entry, identify whether the feared event is occurring presently or is anticipated in the future. Then, over the next days, record whether that feared event materialized, and if it did, whether it was truly as intolerable as expected. This exercise will help you avoid wasting too much of your present moments fearing something that often never occurs.

Begin the habit—at the close of each day—of offering gratitude for having gotten through another day. This repeated practice helps us focus our attention on the day at hand and develop an appreciation for living life with greater consciousness and intent.

SIX

TRANSFORMING NEGATIVITY INTO POSITIVE EMOTIONS AND ACTIONS

Key characteristics of the people who transformed their lives through illness or disability were their ability and determination to turn negativity into positive emotions and actions. Many expressed that it would have been easy for them to become imprisoned by pity for themselves or frozen in inactivity by fear or sadness. Instead, they made a concerted effort to remain positive about their lives and their opportunities to make a difference in the lives of others. These people truly desired to use what illness or disability had taught them to help other people; they were determined that something good would come out of their experience. In their effort to create a positive environment in which to live, they sought out optimistic others—others who remained steadfast in their positive outlook on life, who spoke positively, who acted positively, and who gently encouraged others to do the same.

The people interviewed for this book who made positive thinking and acting a daily practice often learned to catch their own negative thoughts and to challenge the validity of those thoughts. In turn, they tried to act on their positive thoughts rather than allowing negativity to pervade their interactions with others and themselves. Some expressed a belief that positive energy attracts positive energy, and they used this belief to attract the healing energy they needed to survive whatever situations they encountered. Others equated maintaining a positive attitude with hope—hope that they could find meaning in their illness, hope that they could use what they had learned to help others, hope that they could continue to experience life with the quality and satisfaction that make life livable. (See "Further Reading" for resources on healing.)

Beth's Use of Illness to Change Negative Thoughts and Behaviors

Beth was a 45-year-old family physician who had been married for 20 years and had two teenage children. Last summer Beth was rushed to the emergency ward of her hospital when she began experiencing severe tightness in her chest and arms and an inability to catch her breath. At only 45, Beth was experiencing a heart attack. Fortunately, because of her medical training, she accurately identified her symptoms and received the medical attention necessary to save her life. Although Beth had a family history of heart disease, she was nevertheless shocked by her cardiac condition. Her only risk factor had been an elevated cholesterol level, which was being treated.

I NEVER SMOKED, I ATE HEALTHILY, I exercised every day. I was the healthiest person I knew when I had my heart attack. I was completely taken aback by what happened to me. My father died of heart disease but at age 62, and he had been a heavy smoker. I knew that my family history put me at risk, but I really never thought I'd actually have a heart attack. I was terrified, and so was my family. To think that I could have died. To be so close to death and have it all end. This experience changed me. It's changed the way I interact with my family, my patients, even the way I act toward myself.

I think it began several years ago, when I had a cyst in my left breast. It was in the left lower quadrant, and I knew that breast cancer is often in the right outer quadrant. So I knew it wasn't breast cancer. The spot was right in front of my heart. And I really believe now that it was my anger. I had taken all of my anger and projected it into this cyst right by my heart. For years I knew that I was holding onto a lot of anger. I was angry at my husband for never considering my feelings in the decisions we made. I was angry at my two kids for not appreciating what I was working so hard to give them. And I was angry at my mother and my sisters for expecting so much from me and giving very little in return. I think that I felt hurt—that the love I had given had been rejected. Or maybe even that I was unlovable to the people I loved the most. And I think that the years of anger manifested into a mass in my breast, right over my heart.

I've come to believe that my heart attack came about in a similar manner—that it happened because of the negative way I was reacting to how my life was turning out. Even the term *heart attack*—it's an attack on the heart, on the ability to love and feel loved. All of my life I worried about the future. I worried about how my kids were going to turn out. I worried about my marriage. I worried about whether my practice would be successful. And all of my life I've had intense negative reactions to things and people. I see this now as stemming from my own feelings about myself—my own inability to accept myself fully and to believe that I was worthy of being accepted by others. So I would project that negativity onto others and see them as negative, before others had the chance to project it onto me. This way if I felt rejected by them, I could reject them first.

Well, I learned that I was setting myself up for rejection by doing this. And after my heart attack, I made a conscious decision to stop living this way. So I disciplined myself to stop this kind of negative thinking. I had to bring these thoughts to a conscious level and make myself become aware of my negative thoughts when I had them. In other words, when I had these negative reactions or emotions about people or things, I had to recognize them for what they were, instead of allowing them to run me—to determine my reactions. It's seeing the glass as half empty as opposed to half full. I always saw the glass as half empty until my kids started doing this. And I realized that I had probably taught them to do this. And it made me stop and rethink my own perspective about things, my own reactions. I asked myself, "Why am I always so negative?" I think it was because I felt insecure and afraid. And then I had to examine why I felt insecure and afraid. And a lot of it came down to feeling unacceptable and unlovable. I realized that I was projecting these feelings onto the external world so that everything and everyone else became unacceptable and unlovable instead of me. That was a real revelation for me.

I realized also that I was trying to control not only my life but my husband's and my kids' lives. I was afraid because my kids were getting older and I didn't like some of the decisions they were making about their lives. I was afraid for them, because I thought that they were making bad decisions that would hurt them and their opportunities to have a better life. And I was afraid of seeing them get hurt. Even though I know that everyone has to learn from their own mistakes, it's still painful to see your children get hurt because of the decisions they make.

I realized that I was attached to my fear and attached to the idea that my kids should turn out well and that I should make sure of this. After my heart attack, I let go of this attachment. I let go of trying to control my kids' lives, and instead I let them make their own mistakes. I try to practice a greater detachment from involving myself in their decisions. I try to allow them the freedom to make their own decisions and live with the consequences. I've stopped giving them direction unless it has to do with safety and health issues. Otherwise, I've learned that they have the right to make their own decisions and to learn from them. They have to learn that they have choices, and I can't make these choices for them. I realized that my kids were interpreting my advice as criticism and judgment. And when I stopped giving advice that felt critical to them, we all started getting along a lot better. It was just easier to be together. There wasn't this constant conflict anymore. I think I learned how to be with my kids without judging them and their decisions. And that allowed us to be together and feel comfortable.

I also had to come to terms with my disappointment that my marriage did not turn out exactly as I expected. It's been hard trying to make this relationship work; we've gone through a lot together, and I think we've hurt each other over the years. I'm trying to learn to be more accepting of Bill and less demanding that he be someone he's not. Bill is a thinking person, and I'm a feeling person. So we don't communicate using the same language, and we don't interpret specific situations in the same way. And when I started understanding that this is who he is and how he perceives things, I could let go of the idea that he was doing things to purposely hurt me. It always felt to me like he wasn't considering my feelings. And I used to be very angry about that. I felt betrayed and hurt. Now I realize that this is who he is. He's not as sensitive as me. He can't as easily put himself into another's shoes and understand how his behaviors may hurt me or the kids. But I realize now that he hasn't meant to hurt me. He made decisions without realizing how I'd react.

I've come to realize also that I'm responsible for making myself happy. I can't expect someone else to make me happy. I can't depend on or expect my husband or my kids to do this for me. And it's not my responsibility to make sure that they're happy either. So I no longer have the expectation that we should all be one big, happy family. How we are is how we are, and that's OK. Now I make sure that I take responsibility for bringing enjoyment to my day. If I'm having a hard day, I do something to make the pressure lighter. I won't go home in a bad mood and expect my family to make me feel better. That's just looking for disaster. I've learned that when I treat myself with kindness and do things to make me feel good, then the pressure is not on my family to do this—and we all get along better.

I think that what I learned from my heart attack is how much I was creating negativity in my life and how I didn't have to live this way. For a long time I blamed my husband and my kids for my heart attack. And then I realized that they didn't cause anything; I allowed myself to feel let down, hurt, unloved. And that was my choice—it wasn't necessarily the reality of how things were. And I didn't have to perceive things this way. It was my choice to see the glass as half empty instead of half full.

My choices are different today. Whenever I start getting frustrated with my kids or with my husband or with difficult patients, I try to remember that I could have died and that I'm lucky to be here now. And that single thought allows me to feel that whatever it is I'm concerned about in the moment doesn't really matter. What matters is that I have this chance right now to choose to see the good in the situation, to let go of my need to control it, to let go of my fear about it, and to be thankful for the love that is in my life, instead of ignoring it or judging it to be unacceptable because it doesn't meet my expectations.

I also learned that I can make choices about whom I want to spend my time with. I grew up in a very judgmental family. And I learned to be the same way. Today, I try to surround myself with people—mostly friends—who are open-minded and accepting. Because it feels good to be with such people. I feel their acceptance, and I want to give that acceptance to others. I don't want to spend my time anymore with people who are closed-minded and very critical, because it doesn't feel good. It makes me uncomfortable, and I feel judged. And now that I know the difference between what it feels like to be with people who are open and accepting and what it feels like to be with people who are hypercritical and judgmental, I can make the choice to be with friends who are positive in their outlook and who help me to stay positive, too.

Exercise 1: Identifying Negative Self-talk

All action stems from thought. The way we think about our world determines how we interact with it. Our thoughts directly influence our experiences. It is important to recognize, however, that what happens in life is, of itself, neutral. We decide whether we perceive our experience as positive or negative. We judge and impose our own meaning on every experience we encounter.

It is necessary to inspect how our experience of the world is directly related to our judgment and interpretation. We must first begin with an examination of the continuous stream of consciousness that courses through our mind—our own self-talk. *Self-talk* is the voice in our mind that offers a running commentary on all of our experience. We commonly develop our self-talk based on the style of interaction with which we were raised. In Chapter 5 you identified whether you grew up in a background characterized by critical judgment or acceptance.

Take 15 minutes and examine the self-talk that emerges naturally in your mind in response to events in your environment. Write your self-talk down on paper so that you can better understand the patterns that emerge. Ask yourself these questions:

❦ Is your self-talk hypercritical, judging, or fearful? Our self-talk reflects the relationship we have with ourselves, whether we treat ourselves with compassion and gentleness or with harshness and exacting standards.

❦ What does your self-talk indicate about the relationship you have with yourself? How do you typically treat yourself as you go about your day?

❦ Does your self-talk reflect optimism or pessimism?

❦ Do you hold yourself to perfectionistic standards that are unrealistic or unattainable?

If you find that your self-talk is harsher than you realized, practice talking to yourself with greater gentleness, compassion, and acceptance. When you make a mistake, instead of responding with critical, condemning self-talk, stop and remind yourself that mistakes are part of the process of growth in all human lives and that, without mistakes, we would have no opportunity to grow and change for the better. Use mindfulness training to catch all self-condemning thoughts, such as, "I'm so stupid, I can't believe I did that" or "Only an idiot would have made such an error." When you experience self-condemning thoughts, stop and substitute more self-loving and accepting thoughts, such as "Everyone makes mistakes" and "I can stop beating myself up for this mistake and instead see what I can do to correct things."

Mindfulness training helps us catch our negative thoughts and challenge them. It is important, however, to understand that the goal is not simply to substitute negative thoughts with positive ones; the goal is to catch our negative thoughts and challenge their validity. When we can understand that our negative thoughts are too harsh, then we can begin to modify them using thoughts that encourage greater forgiveness of ourselves.

Simply substituting negative thoughts with positive ones will not help us make permanent changes in our style of self-talk. Unless we truly believe the positive thoughts we are substituting, our behaviors will remain fear-based and hypercritical. A better method to bring about permanent change is to recognize that our style of self-talk is damaging, to challenge our condemning self-judgments, and to make small modifications in our self-talk style over time.

Exercise 2: Releasing Negativity From Our Hearts

To heal, we must release negative emotions from our hearts. But to release negative emotions, we must first become aware of such feelings. To do this, we must acknowledge our feelings of inadequacy, our fears, our mistakes, our anger, and our sadness. If we deny or do not express such emotions, they can make us both emotionally and physically sick.

In your journal, identify your feelings of inadequacy. Acknowledge that all people have feelings of inadequacy and that such feelings are a normal part of being human. We commonly feel proficient in certain life skills and lacking in others. In what areas of your life do you feel inadequate? Can you determine where these feelings stem from? Can you remember the first time that you felt inadequate in each area? Have there been periods in your life when you felt a greater sense of proficiency? If so, what characterized these periods?

Ask the same questions about your fears; mistakes; and feelings of guilt, anger, and sadness. Remember, all of these feelings are normal and shared by every human being who ever existed. The goal is not to chastise yourself for having these feelings but rather to allow them to surface in your consciousness so that they do not emerge in unconscious ways that cause sickness or conflict in your life. Only when they are consciously experienced can these emotions be healed and released.

It is important that we do not view these emotions as bad. Anger, sadness, guilt, and fear are not bad in and of themselves, and we are not bad for experiencing them. They are part of the gamut of human emotions, and we all experience them to one degree or another. To attempt to never experience them again is probably impossible. We will always experience fear, inadequacy, guilt, anger, and sadness. We will continue to make mistakes as long as we live. To believe otherwise is to hold ourselves to unattainable, inhuman standards—standards that can bring only disappointment and feelings of failure.

Our goal is to acknowledge these emotions and to forgive ourselves for them—to understand that we are still OK even though we experience them. Our goal is to heal these emotions, not to believe that we must never experience them again. But once we have acknowledged the presence of these emotions in our hearts, it is then necessary to do the following:

🕊 Ask yourself if you truly must hold on to these feelings. Are your fears founded? If they are not, why are you allowing them to govern your life? If your fears are founded, what good does it do to waste the present moment fearing something that will occur in the future?

🕊 If you are still angry, ask yourself what purpose your anger serves. How is it benefiting you to hold on to your anger?

🕊 Do you experience guilt? Have you expressed your guilt and attempted to make amends to those you believe you harmed? We commonly feel guilt for past mistakes that we continue to hold ourselves accountable for, long after such feelings have finished facilitating our growth. We may even continue to harshly blame ourselves for past infractions that were never as injurious as we perceived. Such misconstrued guilt only reinforces notions of our unworthiness.

🕊 Are you still experiencing grief and sadness over your illness or other past losses? If so, you must examine whether your sadness is preventing you from moving forward in your life and creating a daily existence in which you find meaning and can positively contribute to others' lives.

Recognize that it is time to release these feelings from your heart. They no longer need to be your ball and chain. Sometimes we hold on to old emotions because they have become familiar and comfortable, even if they do not serve our greater growth. It is always frightening to relinquish that which is known and comfortable. However, to heal, we must take the risk of stepping into the unknown.

To release inharmonious emotions, the Buddhists practice acting in opposition to emotions they wish to abandon. (See "Further Reading" for resources on Buddhism.) If we are sad, we should make an effort to engage in activity that will lighten our hearts and particularly the hearts of others, because bringing joy to others is the most direct way to lighten our own souls. If we are fearful, we must take a risk and engage in the activity we fear. We must do the same for our feelings of anger and guilt. In your journal, record how you felt when you acted in direct opposition to your inharmonious emotions. Assess to what degree your actions alleviated the feelings you were seeking to release.

It is also important to recognize whether we feel broken or wounded as a result of our illness. We may experience these feelings at a level of consciousness we can barely detect. But if we harbor feelings that we are irreparably damaged by illness or disability, such feelings will influence our perceptions about our experience, often on an unconscious level. We must recognize that, even while we are physically ill, we can remain spiritually whole—that our wholeness as a human being is not affected by physical illness or disability unless we allow it. When we allow both to affect our spirit, we lose hope that life can be maintained at a quality worth living. This is usually when disease fastens its grasp.

It is important to ask yourself if you view your illness or disability as a punishment. If you do, examine why you feel you are being punished. Are such emotions related to feelings of guilt that you identified above? Who is punishing you, and for what reason? Do you feel that you deserve to be punished? Often we feel that we are being punished when we can find no other reason for our suffering—when our pain seems to be unjust and when it has no clear purpose in our lives. But feelings of punishment inappropriately reinforce fears that we are unworthy and bad. We must challenge such feelings and understand them as our own effort to make sense out of a seemingly senseless event. It is helpful to attempt to create sense out of our illness or disability, but we grow only if we do this in a positive way—for example, by finding reasons why we needed this particular life lesson. Ask yourself what you have learned from your illness or disability that you would not have otherwise known. Try to identify how some form of good could come from your suffering and loss.

Do you feel sorry for yourself? Do these feelings prevent you from creating a livable life, enjoying the small satisfactions present in your daily existence and finding value in each day? Feelings of self-pity commonly trap us in states of inaction. If you feel frozen by self-pity, it is important to first acknowledge this emotion. Remember that if we deny our feelings, we often release them unconsciously in the form of attacks against those close to us. Recognize that resentment and self-pity are normal human emotions and that you are OK for experiencing them. Do not berate or condemn yourself for having these feelings. But recognize also that such feelings are likely preventing you from living as fully as possible.

To begin to release self-pity, practice acting in opposition to this emotion. Participate in activities that demonstrate that you are grateful for your life. Often we best display gratitude by giving to others; giving to others demonstrates our appreciation for the riches we have received. Identify two ways that you can give to others in the next three weeks. Select activities that are simple and do not require a great deal of energy if you have little to spare. Often, mundane activities that we tend to overlook are the most appreciated by people in need. For example, we could prepare a meal for another, shop for someone who cannot get to the store, or telephone a person who is frequently home alone.

Exercise 3: Turning Negativity Into Positive Experience

People who have used illness to positively transform their lives state that illness taught them to make the best of seeming misfortune. Transforming a negative event into a positive situation is a difficult life skill that requires disciplined practice over lengthy periods. It involves resourcefulness, creativity, the ability to visualize a positive outcome, and the identification of ways of enabling that positive outcome to materialize. It also involves the capacity to maintain the hope that good can come from seemingly distressful life circumstances.

In the past, have you been able to find positive experience in the midst of a negative situation? Record the following in your journal:

🖎 Identify the life situations in your past in which you were able to create something positive from a disturbing event. Examine the methods you used to accomplish this task. Were you able to summon strengths and skills that you did not realize you possessed? Identify these specific strengths and skills, and determine if you have continued to develop them throughout your life. How can you use these strengths and skills in your present situation to alleviate your suffering?

🖎 Identify three ways in which you can create a positive outcome from your present struggle. Identify small, simple actions, and record them in your journal. Writing these on paper will strengthen your commitment to materializing them in your daily life.

🖎 Can you help another person who has just begun to experience the illness that you have been living with? Can you help that person better understand what to expect and share strategies to manage the illness that only an experienced person would know?

🖎 Can you use your illness to become closer to your loved ones? Perhaps your illness has offered you the opportunity to express your tenderness and gratitude to those closest to you. Has it deepened the intimacy and trust you feel for these people? Can you make the effort to communicate your feelings directly, recognizing that you might have missed this opportunity if illness did not provide the impetus?

❦ Has your illness encouraged you to establish healthy lifestyle changes that could serve as a positive model for your younger loved ones, such as quitting smoking, eating less junk food and exercising more, and maintaining a positive attitude in the face of challenge?

Exercise 4: Surrounding Ourselves With Positive People

Ultimately, the responsibility for engaging in and sustaining positive actions and speech in our lives lies with us. No one can transform our negative experience into a positive event for us. The interactions we maintain with others, however, can influence our effort to preserve life-affirming behaviors in the face of challenge.

It is important to ask yourself if your relationships feel positive or negative. Generally, people know whether a specific relationship feels supportive and compassionate or draining and hypercritical. Ask yourself if the primary relationships in your life feel good to you. It is important to consider each relationship separately. Is each relationship characterized by understanding, gentleness, and compassion? Or do you commonly feel drained after being with a particular person? Do you spend a good deal of time defending your actions and desires to that individual? Are you offered unsolicited advice that implies that you cannot take care of yourself and that someone else knows what you need better than you do? Relationships characterized by the latter qualities deplete our energy, particularly when illness has already lowered our energy levels.

When we are in crisis or are attempting to make life-affirming changes, it is important to surround ourselves with positive people—people who are both respectful of our desire to enact change and who understand how to offer the emotional support we need. It is our responsibility, however, to learn how to ask for the kind of emotional support that feels good to us. Often we do not directly ask for this support, instead assuming that others can read our minds or innately perceive our needs better than we can communicate.

The assumption that others (especially our loved ones) can offer the emotional support we need without our assistance is false. We must learn to ask for the kind of love and compassion we desire, while recognizing that people have different ways of demonstrating love and may be earnestly trying to do so for us. Many people have not learned how to be emotionally supportive in a way that feels positive rather than disapproving. People who grew up in an environment characterized by anger, judgment, and attack find it very difficult to demonstrate compassion in a style other than criticism. Try to recognize that these people are doing the best they can; they may not even recognize how harsh their interactions feel to you. In your efforts to ask for support that feels positive, remember not to take offense or to attack others. Instead, practice asking for what you need in a loving way, and offer others the opportunity to communicate their needs. Recognize also that witnessing your illness may likely trigger fears about loss in others.

If an emotionally unsupportive relationship is not valuable to you, then consider removing yourself from that interaction. It is important to recognize, however, that when we pull away from others, we are closing off opportunities for companionship and love. If we are unable to find compassion in a relationship, it is probably best to reconsider whether we want to continue exposing ourselves to that level of negativity.

Do not allow yourself to be affected by others' negativity. Frequently, when we spend time with others who are angry, critical, and rejecting, we tend to be influenced by that kind of negativity, sometimes unconsciously. That is why it is so critical to surround ourselves with others who are steadfast in their positive actions and speech. Not only does being around positive people reinforce our own practice of such behaviors, but their positive energy influences our emotional state. For this reason we often find that we feel better after spending time with people who act in loving and compassionate ways.

When we cannot avoid spending time with people who act and speak negatively, we must remember that such negativity belongs to them—not to us. Rather than allowing their pessimism to affect our mood, we must consciously choose not to participate in the negative aspects of the interaction. It is unfruitful to respond to others' negativity with anger, a critical attack, or demands for change. Maintaining our emotional equanimity in the midst of interaction with a negative person requires that we accept this person's need for negativity but refuse to participate in it. Instead, the Buddhists suggest that the best way to deal with another's negativity is to respond with compassion and to remember that negativity stems from feelings of insecurity that are projected. (See "Further Reading" for resources on Buddhism.)

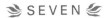

SEVEN

UNDERSTANDING AND LETTING GO OF THE ILLUSION OF CONTROL

Joseph Campbell, the renowned mythologist, observed that none of us live the lives we intend. (See "Further Reading" for resources on mythology and the lessons of human life.) Instead, our lives unfold in ways we never planned. Our best-laid plans are commonly shattered by events over which we have no control. The people who found meaning through illness or disability spoke of the need to release the illusion that life can be controlled and to realize that the only thing that can be controlled in human life is the way we respond to crisis. They expressed that the control we have lies in our perspective—how we choose to view the events that unfold in our lives and whether we choose to view our hardships as opportunities for growth or as senseless events. These people were adamant that the key to their own self-empowerment was the realization that their sense of control lay in their own perspective and not in anything external to themselves. And it came when they relinquished the illusion of control for a more realistic understanding of what they could and could not change.

Megan's Experience Living With the Uncertainty of Illness and Letting Go of Control

Megan was a 50-year-old nurse who worked in a neonatal intensive care unit. She was divorced and had two adult children living in different parts of the country. In adolescence Megan was diagnosed with juvenile diabetes, and as she aged, she experienced significant medical complications of the disease—diabetic retinopathy, neuropathy in her lower limbs, and frozen shoulder syndrome. Megan also had been in remission from ovarian cancer for one year. Although the treatment for her cancer appeared to have been effective, the radiation and chemotherapy exacerbated her diabetes-related medical conditions. Some days it was difficult for Megan to walk. She was forced to stop driving because of her worsening visual problems and neuropathy. And she did not know how much longer she could continue to work as a nurse.

WHEN I WAS 14, I WAS TOLD that I had juvenile diabetes. My grandfather also had juvenile diabetes, and he died pretty young, maybe 50—people in those days didn't live very long with the disease. The medical profession didn't really understand it; they didn't know what they were doing. So I was diagnosed at a time when there wasn't very good medical care for the disease. There were no meters to test your blood sugar levels—they had urine sticks instead—so I was supposed to monitor my urinary sugar levels. I had a diet that was so restrictive that it was impossible even for someone who was highly motivated to stay on it. I was on one shot of insulin a day, which was not very effective at regulating my sugar levels, and I was constantly up and down. Feeling good, and then crashing—all day long.

And people would tell me horror stories about all of the people who had diabetes they knew who didn't take care of themselves and died or went blind—like the girl who lived down the street and went blind because she was a diabetic and ate candy. It was really pretty awful, the stories people told me, thinking that this was a good way to motivate someone to take care of themselves.

I also grew up in a family with an alcoholic father. We were five kids, and my mother stayed at home. She tried her best, but I think she was pretty depressed herself. The really hard thing was growing up with my father. I don't ever remember a time when he wasn't drinking since I was a very small child. He didn't stop drinking until after I moved out of their home. I think that as a child, I had to develop ways to cope with my father's alcoholism. I don't have a lot of memories of when I was young, but in our bedroom we used to have a closet. And I remember spending a lot of time in that closet, crying. I spent a lot of my young childhood hoping that someone would rescue me, that someone would just come and take me, or that I'd get hit by a car.

And I learned that the way to manage in life was to really try to please other people. I think that I thought—I think all of my brothers and sisters thought—that if we were really good children, my father would stop drinking, that we would have a family like everybody else if we were really good. So I became a really good kid. I was a good student, I helped my mother, I was sweet and polite. I tried to do whatever I was expected to do; I tried to be very good, to behave very well, not to cause any problems. I understand now that as a child I was trying to find some control over life because it seemed to be very much out of control.

When I became an adult, there were better medical interventions to manage diabetes, but it's a disease that can be difficult to control. So I spent most of my adult years trying earnestly to do what I was supposed to do as a diabetic. I tried to eat right, I tested my blood sugars regularly, I exercised to stay in good health. But even with all of my efforts to do everything right, I still experienced diabetes-related complications. And that was discouraging. I'd have these periods when I'd feel so discouraged that I'd eat horribly or I wouldn't test my sugars. And then I'd feel worse, so I'd go back to rigidly following the prescribed dietary regulations. It was like being on a roller coaster for many years.

Then, two years ago, I was diagnosed with ovarian cancer, which was a real shock. It was as if somebody punched me. I thought, "This can't be. Haven't I experienced enough between growing up with an alcoholic father and having diabetes since I was a kid?" I was so angry. I had always done all of the right things to avoid cancer and to take care of myself. It doesn't run in my family; I ate right, I didn't smoke, and I didn't drink. So I thought, "Well, what else could I have possibly done to prevent it?" And that's when I first realized how much I always tried to control my life and that in reality we truly don't have control over very much of life.

For a while I blamed God for the diabetes and the cancer. By the time I was a teenager, I had stopped going to church, and over the years I had become very angry at whatever belief I had in God. And that took a lot of time to work on, before I realized that God didn't give me the diabetes or the cancer, that disease is something that just happens in life. It took a long time before I could understand that I wasn't being punished.

For some reason, in this society we don't really expect bad things to happen. We have these fairy-tale expectations. I don't know if it's this society or just part of being human. But I know that in some other cultures you're raised with the idea that life is not always going to go as you planned; in fact, life mostly doesn't go as we plan or hope. Before the cancer I never realized how much I sought to control my life. I really believed that if I did things the way they were supposed to be done and I followed the rules, then things would turn out the way I hoped. And through several disappointing things in my life—the diabetes, growing up with an alcoholic father, the difficulty I had with my two pregnancies, my divorce, the cancer—I realized that there's only so much that's under our control, and most things that happen in life are beyond our control. And that's just the way it is. Life went out of control in my childhood and adolescence, and ever since I've been fighting furiously to get it back—only to realize that I can't control it. Life can't be controlled. It's easier to accept it as it happens and deal with it day by day.

I spent a lot of time thinking about why this happened, and why me, and how awful it was. And as I said, for a while I blamed God. It took a tremendous amount of energy trying to figure it all out. I don't know why the illnesses happened. But once I came to the realization that God didn't send this to me—that no one sent this to me—I was able to channel my energy in directions that were more positive. When I gave up the idea that I had to figure it out and get control over it, I freed up a lot of energy and time to do more constructive things. Giving up the need to have control over my illnesses allowed me to start figuring out how I could live with them and still have a quality of life that was satisfactory to me.

What helped me the most was to better understand what I could control and what I couldn't, instead of thinking that I should be able to control everything. For years I would set up such rigid expectations for myself as a diabetic that I just couldn't meet them. And then I'd get really upset with myself; I'd feel like a failure and then give up. What helped me was giving up those expectations and instead working on one little piece of my care so that I wasn't constantly setting myself up for failure. I learned that I do best when I set goals for my care that are small, reasonable, doable things that need to get done. Even with the cancer, I had so much to do—getting information, choosing a doctor, choosing a method of treatment, going to a support group—that I felt overwhelmed and out of control. I felt that the cancer had taken control of my life. So I said, "OK, what can I do to realistically help myself?" So every day I'd make one or two telephone calls and appointments until I was able to get at least some things done each day and feel that I had some control over what was happening. I had to start understanding and respecting my limitations—that I could do only so much in a day before I felt fatigued, that I could take in only so much information before I felt overwhelmed, that I could make only so many decisions in a day.

It also was very important for me to let go of the idea that I had to do everything about my care perfectly. It's only been very recently that I've been able to say, "I'm a person with diabetes and cancer and I am who I am, I do what I can do. And if I don't do it perfectly, it's really OK." I'm not a failure if I didn't do it well enough today—if I missed an appointment because I didn't feel well, or if I didn't eat right today. I think that's been really important for me—to learn not to hold onto failures, to stop beating myself up for not being perfect. And to know that tomorrow I can always try to take care of myself better than I was able to today. It's OK that I don't have control over everything I want to about my illnesses. The Serenity Prayer has become very meaningful to me—to be able to tell the difference between what I can and cannot control and to be able to accept what's out of my control. (See "Further Reading" for resources on the Serenity Prayer.)

I learned from these experiences that we really can't control anything but our own decisions and attitudes. That's the one thing that I can control—the decisions I make, given the options that I have available, and the attitude I have about what's happening. Once I let go of my need to control everything and stopped beating myself up for feeling like a failure, it was like a weight was lifted off me. The cancer has become another chronic disease for me to live with. In some ways, being a diabetic has made living with cancer easier, because I already knew how to live with one chronic illness. Now there are more appointments, more things to do, more medicine, more treatments, but it's all kind of the same. And my attitude has changed. I no longer need to figure out why my illnesses happened to me or to have control over them. I do what's in my power to manage my care. I try to make informed decisions to the best of my ability. Beyond that, I've let go of the need to do everything perfectly to control it. I do what I can each day and try to live one day at a time. And I've found that that's the best way for me to live with the uncertainty of illness.

Exercise 1: Identifying Our Belief in the Illusion of Control

What is the illusion of control? It is an invention that people, throughout time, have created to live more comfortably with the uncertainty of life. It involves the idea that we can con- duct our lives in a way that lessens the likelihood of hardship.

All of us participate in this illusion, whether by purchasing insurance, carrying charms to bring luck, or repeating positive affirmations. Many of us believe that, if we do all of the right things—things we were told to do by people we held as authority figures—we can avoid adversity. Many of us also find out the hard way that this belief is merely an illusion. We may eat healthy foods and exercise, but we become ill despite these efforts. We may seek an education and work hard and still find ourselves unemployed in a recession. Or we may strive to be a good person, obeying every civil and religious law we were taught, and still endure trauma we never imagined. Examine the beliefs you have held about your ability to control life circumstances and the ways you have sought control over your life.

🖐 Have you believed that you could reduce the occurrence of misfortune by doing everything you were told by authority figures? Examine how this belief has influenced the decisions you have made throughout your life.

🖐 Did you come from a family background in which the illusion of control was taught either overtly or covertly? Did your parents attempt to exert control over your life or their own?

Many people who lived through traumatic historical events—most recently, the Great Depression, World War II, and the Holocaust—were forced to construct lives amid great instability and uncertainty. To prevent their children from living with the same insecurity, many tried to shape their children's lives to ensure greater stability and certainty. Although the generation that experienced these events understood that life truly could not be controlled, their children, who grew up in the relative calm and prosperity of the 1950s and early 1960s, were more predisposed to accept the illusion of control. At various times in their lives, this generation, the baby boomers, has alternately rebelled against and accepted the idea that life can be controlled by behaving in accordance with established social norms.

If you are a member of this generation, you may need to pay particular attention to your belief in the illusion of control and the extent to which this belief has operated in your life. It also is necessary to examine whether you are seeking to exert control over your life—and your illness—in the present. We often try to exert control when our safety is threatened. The experience of illness commonly undermines our sense of safety by evoking primitive fears of dependency and helplessness. Ask yourself if you feel that your safety has been threatened by illness. It also may be helpful to explore the sense of safety you experienced in childhood. Did you have a childhood in which you felt safe? Or was it marked by frequent change or trauma? Those of us who experienced childhoods that felt unsafe often carry these feelings into adulthood. Such feelings can propel our search for security at all costs. For example, we may have chosen spouses and careers based on our need for security rather than our emotions and natural proclivities. We may search for cures through unsupported treatment methods out of a fear of powerlessness and eventual death. Ask yourself if you are making decisions in the present based on your fears about safety.

Stop and assess whether your safety is truly threatened in the present moment. Often, our sense of threat emerges from fear about an uncertain future rather than from anything that is occurring right now. We worry about our future safety, but our immediate safety is not truly jeopardized. Ask yourself if your safety is genuinely threatened in the present moment. If it is not, you may be causing yourself anxiety without reason.

Exercise 2: Recognizing What We Can and Cannot Realistically Control

Relinquishing the illusion of control requires that we better understand what we can and cannot realistically control. It is first necessary to acknowledge the things we have little or no control over. For example, we cannot control others' behaviors and emotions. We are unable to alter the genetic inheritance that may predispose our bodies and minds to certain illnesses. We cannot foresee and then prevent the occurrence of life events such as accidents, unemployment, and the death of loved ones. We have no command over world events—war, natural disasters, political events—or how these affect our daily life conditions. Explore the following:

🖋 Acknowledge the events and circumstances in your life over which you have no control, and list them in your journal. Have you attempted to exert control over these circumstances in the past? How did these efforts influence your well-being and your relationships with others?

🖋 Generally, our attempt to control others (even when we think it is in their best interest) results in conflict and broken trust. Ask yourself if your attempt to exert control over others was worth the toll taken on you and your loved ones.

🖋 Can you accept the things in your life over which you have no control? Can you allow them to unfold in their own natural course without your intervention? Remember the Buddhist suggestion that the more we seek control over life, the less control we have. (See "Further Reading" for resources on Buddhism.) Control, like much of life, is paradoxical. Just when we think we have our lives under control and on course, an unexpected event occurs to disrupt our well-constructed plans.

It is even more important to recognize what we *do* have control over. Two things we always control are our perspective and the choices we make. Our perspective—whether we see the glass as half empty or half full—influences our experience of the world. We decide how we choose to interpret life circumstances. For example, consider how you view your illness. Is illness a senseless event that has deterred you from the plan you had for your life? Is it a punishment from an angry God—has illness occurred as retribution for sins you committed that seem unforgivable? Or can you believe that your illness occurred to provide you with the life lessons you need to grow spiritually? The perspective that we choose determines whether we see ourselves as a victim of life circumstances or as a participant in life events that facilitate our learning. In your journal, describe your perspective regarding your illness or disability and its meaning in your life.

We also maintain control over our choices about participation in specific events and relationships. It is always our decision whether we wish to continue activities and relationships that do not feel supportive of our needs. Even if the choices available to us are not to our liking, we must recognize that choices *are* available and that *we* determine how we perceive our options. When we perceive our options as unacceptable, however, we should remember that, from our present vantage point, we are often unable to understand a particular situation's potential value in our life. Using the adage about one door closing and another opening, when a much-desired door closes in our lives, we often experience pain and confusion. It is only later, when another opens—one that leads to greater growth experiences—that we begin to understand why we had to endure the pain that occurred when the first door closed.

❧ Use your journal to examine the choices you have available in your present life circumstances. Consider how you perceive these options and whether you may benefit by broadening your perception.

❧ Assess whether your perspective of your current life options has focused on short-term gains and immediate satisfaction. If so, reconsider what your options may include when viewed within your life's broader plan.

We also maintain control over how we choose to respond to the events and people in our environment. Although we may not be able to control the emotions we experience in response to events, we do have control over how we express these emotions. To control how we express our emotions to others, however, we must discipline ourselves to resist acting impulsively on our first emotions. Do you react to situations without reflecting first, or have you learned to explore your initial reactions slowly and deliberately before you act on them? If you tend to express your emotions abruptly, practice nonaction for one full day.

❧ Contemplate each event and examine your emotions in response to it. If others demand that you reply immediately, express that you need a day (or more) to thoroughly consider how you will respond. Assure them that you will address their concerns in the next few days. Record these events in your journal for one week.

❧ Describe the emotions you experienced in the immediate moment. After a day has passed, observe if and how your emotions have changed.

❧ Compare the difference between how you would have reacted in the moment and how you eventually responded after contemplating the situation at greater length.

It is also important to remember that, although we always maintain control over the choices we make, we also have the option to choose differently if we discover that our past decisions are no longer comfortable or workable in our present lives. If we regret choices we made in the past, we can always choose differently in the present. We also can choose to refrain from berating ourselves for past decisions that did not work out as planned and to instead recognize that we made the best decision we could at that time in our lives. Examine the initial choices you made about how you want to live with illness or disability on a daily basis.

🍂 Are these choices still comfortable for you today?

🍂 Do you want to adjust the paths you have taken to deal with your illness or disability?

🍂 Do you desire to make changes in the way you wish to live each day?

Again, identifying and recording specific desires for change (and simple methods of implementation) in your journal will help you maintain your commitment to bring these changes into being. Remember also that the most effective way to change your future is to enact positive change in the present.

Exercise 3: Learning to Live With Uncertainty

Surrendering the illusion of control also requires that we grow more comfortable with uncertainty and our fear of the unknown. Nothing is certain—except that life will present challenges that ask us to stretch our self-imposed limitations to grow. Often life presents us with the opportunity to understand that what we fear most is survivable. We may identify a situation that we fear or believe we cannot endure only to have that very event presented at our door to show us that we can indeed withstand it. Living with uncertainty becomes somewhat easier when we believe that life events occur with a reason—to promote our growth.

One practice that can help us live with uncertainty is to stay focused in the present—to recognize that, most of the time, our safety in the immediate moment is not threatened. We must recognize that our anxiety about survival usually involves some future event that may never happen. Even if that event is certain to happen, we must remember that it is not happening in the immediate moment. If we spend the present worrying about a feared event in the future, we lose the opportunity to make the present moment meaningful now.

 Determine if you are presently experiencing anxiety over an event that will occur in the future. Is the occurrence of this event inevitable and assured?

 Ask yourself if your safety is truly threatened in the immediate moment. If it is not, recognize that you may be missing the opportunity to find satisfaction in the present moment.

 Maintain your focus in the present moment, and decide how you will use it to find meaning and value right now. Identify at least one activity that you can participate in today to bring meaning to the day you are living.

PERCEIVING LIFE AS A SPIRITUAL JOURNEY AND UNDERSTANDING ILLNESS AS PART OF THAT JOURNEY

Many of the people who were able to find meaning through the experience of illness or disability began to perceive their lives as a spiritual journey. They expressed the belief that they are in this world for a purpose and that all things that happen in life occur for a reason. They spoke of receiving guidance through intuition and positive coincidences involving events that seemed to fall into place or that happened at just the right time. They commonly expressed that, through the experience of illness or disability, they began to place their trust in a benevolent universe that promotes their best interests and provides them with what they need to grow on a spiritual path. They expressed that, even though they could not always understand why events occurred, they nevertheless believed that there was meaning in the hardships they endured.

Many also stated that it was important for them to relinquish their need to understand why their illness occurred to accept it and to move past their grief to rebuild their spirit. Some believed that such answers will be given to them when they have completed this life and the lessons learned through this existence. They came to trust that a loving creator has provided the right path and opportunities, even if they do not understand them in the present moment. They learned that it is fruitless to ponder the question "Why did this happen to me?" and instead expressing that a far more fruitful question is "What can I learn from this experience, and how can I use what I've learned to help others?"

Rich's Experience in Finding Deeper Meaning in Seemingly Random Events

When Rich was growing up, he and his family spent two weeks of every summer at their cousins' beach cottage in New Jersey. One summer, when he was 12, Rich got caught in a riptide that pulled him under the ocean's surface. He had always been a strong swimmer, but the powerful current would not release its grip, and Rich could not keep his head above water. There was a storm traveling northward up the coast that day, making the ocean's currents more treacherous. Rich remembers drowning before he was pulled to safety by two lifeguards. The anoxia that he experienced as a result of the depletion of oxygen to his brain for several minutes caused mild brain damage that mirrored the symptoms of a learning disability—lack of ability to focus and concentrate, disorganized thinking, memory problems, and difficulty learning new information. At 68, now a retired businessman who experienced a stroke two years ago, Rich recounted the story of his drowning.

I REMEMBER THE DAY CLEARLY, as though it happened only yesterday. My parents had taken my two brothers and me to the beach, just like every other day. The ocean was a bit more choppy than usual, but the sky was clear blue, and none of us realized that a storm was coming up the coast. I was in the water by myself, not far out at all. I remember that my feet were touching bottom and then suddenly they weren't. I didn't realize that the current had been slowly pulling me farther out into the ocean until the ocean floor dropped off and I wasn't able to touch the bottom anymore. My head went under the water, and I thought that I would swim up to the surface like I always did. But I couldn't. It was as if the ocean were pulling me down, and I couldn't get back to the surface. And I started panicking, desperately trying to bring myself back above the water. It seemed like forever that I was struggling. And then I started getting lightheaded, and it felt like my body had floated upward.

Only I wasn't in my body anymore; I was looking down on my lifeless body in the water. I saw the lifeguards as they lifted my body into their boat and took me back to shore. I saw my parents and my brothers gathered around my body as I lay there on the sand. And then I seemed to travel through a dark tunnel at an exceedingly high speed, until all of a sudden I was with a Being who seemed to emanate an incredible light. I'll never forget this; He put His arms around me and held me. It was the most comforting feeling I've ever felt in my life. And He spoke to me in a voice I'll never forget—I can almost hear it now. He said, "Son, I have plans for you. You're going to be OK." And that's all I remember.

The next thing I knew, I was lying on the sand spitting water out of my lungs, coughing. My mother was crying and holding me. They took me to the local hospital where a doctor checked me over and said that I was fine, that I just needed to rest and get my strength back. But I wasn't fine.

The next weeks were quiet. We had returned to our own home, and my brothers and I counted down the last days we had left before school started—a dreaded ritual we practiced every August until Labor Day came, ending our summer and our freedom. My mother was the only person I told about what happened to me when I drowned. I can still see the shock and awe in her eyes as I told her. She was very quiet, and then she said a prayer thanking God for watching over me.

I remember starting back to school that year thinking things were fine. I was happy to see my friends, and I was excited because it was my first year of junior high and I felt very old and superior to my two younger brothers, who were still in elementary school. But things didn't go so well. It seemed to me that the schoolwork had gotten much harder, which I attributed to being in high school. And my parents told me that I'd just have to work harder, that this wasn't elementary school anymore. So I tried. But no matter how much I tried, I just couldn't do the work. I couldn't concentrate or keep my attention focused on anything for very long. Reading had become torture—I couldn't retain anything I read. And it would take me several attempts to read one sentence before I could understand it. But I just kept thinking that all of this was happening because I was in high school now, and the work was much harder than what I had been used to.

I started to hate school. The only things that interested me were sports and the woodworking shop class. To me, the academic work was just stupid, but that was because I was having so much trouble learning—yet no one realized this. No one picked up that my problems in school might have been connected to the anoxia I experienced. The next years were horrible; I was barely getting by in school. My teachers and my parents were angry with me because they thought I wasn't serious enough about my classes. I almost dropped out, but in my last year of high school I had an English teacher who heard about my drowning and recognized that my difficulty in school may have been related to it. She was the first one who ever connected the two situations. And I thank God for her, because I was at a point where I really didn't see any good reason to stay in school. But I think now that she was brought into my life purposely to help me continue with my education.

This English teacher, Mrs. Bukowski, started tutoring me and helping me to use learning techniques to memorize information and better understand what I read. She was the one who really made me believe in myself and my ability to be successful. By the end of the year, I had passed all of my classes, and Mrs. Bukowski helped me apply to several community colleges in the area. Imagine me! Going to college when just a year before I wanted to drop out of school. Even my guidance counselor had told me to go to the vocational school and get a job in the local factory.

Getting into college was hard, too. People kept telling me that I was wasting my time trying to go to college, that I'd never be able to handle the work. And my grades had been so poor that even the community college in my town didn't want to take me. But Mrs. Bukowski knew the dean of admissions at a community college in Philadelphia, and she appealed to him on my behalf, telling him all about what had happened to me and the change I had made in the past year. She convinced him to give me a chance. And by that time a chance was all I wanted. I knew if I had a chance, I could be successful. So I applied, got accepted, and moved to Philadelphia.

I met my wife at this school, and she became my best friend, my soul mate, and my teacher. It was my wife who really helped me finish college in the next years. And by that time I was determined that I wanted to get my bachelor's degree and become an architect. Building things and working with my hands always came easy to me. But again, I got letters of rejection, one after another. It was very humiliating and discouraging, especially because I felt like a failure to my wife. Well, of course, she was wonderful about the situation and kept encouraging me and helping me have the confidence to keep trying. Eventually, though, I decided that enough was enough; I needed to work and have food on the table, for her sake at least.

I got a job in—wouldn't you guess—a local manufacturing plant, a factory. Just the place they said I'd end up. I felt very ashamed, and I thought that I had let my wife down. But she always maintained her confidence in me and kept telling me to be patient—that something good would come of this. Well, all I wanted to do was get out of that job; I was on an assembly line that packaged canned goods. But soon my wife was expecting our first child, and I knew that I had to make a go of this job to provide for her and the baby. I worked hard and was promoted to floor manager. But I hated it, and I felt that I was wasting any skills that I did have.

One day I was driving home when I saw the president of the plant on the side of the road with a flat tire. He didn't know me from Adam, but I stopped and changed the tire for him, and he invited my wife and me over for dinner to thank me. They lived in a beautiful estate in one of the old money neighborhoods outside Philadelphia. During the course of the night, he told me about several plans he and his wife had for renovating their home, and I offered to do the work for him because I needed the money.

I remember feeling pretty despondent after that dinner—that my life was at a dead end and that I would never have a chance to be successful. I'll tell you, it was hard to see how he lived and then go home to our tiny apartment. I felt sorry for myself and sorry for my wife and baby. But in a couple of days, he called me and asked if I could start the construction work we had talked about. I worked almost every weekend for several months from six in the morning to late at night. I often stopped only because I couldn't see anymore once night had come. But I finished the work, and my boss was impressed. He got me jobs on other people's homes, and I began working so much that I had to hire my own help. Soon I left the factory job and started my own construction business.

And in the next years I realized that this is what I was really good at—seeing an idea in my head and creating it with my hands. I did OK in the first few years; nothing spectacular, but I always managed to stay in the black financially. One day my old boss called me. His company was doing well, and he wanted to renovate the old plant and build new office space. He asked me if I wanted the job, not because I had experience renovating factories, he said, but because he respected my skills and knew that I was honest and dependable. I turned him down at first, because I had never built anything that large and I felt that I'd be in over my head. But he assured me that his engineer would work with me and that he was confident that I could handle the job. So I took it.

When I look back, I can see how fortunate I was—how circumstances just fell into place at the right time to help me. I'm not sure that I would have made it through architecture school because of the heavy reading and math. But running my own construction company was something that seemed to come easy to me. And it turned out that the courses I took in college helped me learn the business end of things. I was really lucky that my old boss gave me a chance, that he saw something in me that no one else did, except for maybe my wife. When I think back, this was another instance when someone came into my life at a pivotal period and changed the course of my life.

After I finished my boss's new plant, I started bidding on similar jobs and got several of them. And that's when my business started to take off. In the next years my company expanded, and I became known as a respected builder in the Philadelphia area. When I had a stroke at age 66, I retired from the company after being its president for 34 years—I handed it over to my son. In the last years I was still president, we converted several old warehouses in Philadelphia into residential housing for people who couldn't otherwise afford homes. My son has carried that on, and every year we donate a portion of our revenues to the restoration of deteriorated buildings for residential housing for low-income families.

That was my success story—going from being brain damaged because of drowning to being president of a respected and successful construction company. I was very lucky in my life. People and opportunities came about at just the right moments to help me. I learned that when one door closes, another opens. I've had so many obstacles to overcome because of the brain damage I had from drowning. Sometimes it felt like one thing after another. But I tried to persevere and accomplish what I set out to do. The end goal didn't always end up looking like what I had initially imagined. But I learned that this was OK, too.

You can always say "This is too hard, I'm going to give up." But it's easy to give up. I've been able to look back at the struggles I've been through and appreciate the opportunities I had. And I've come to better understand why certain doors opened for me and why others remained shut; I couldn't understand these things when they were happening at the time. I wouldn't be where I am today if I didn't accept the doors that opened for me, if I had been bent on going through only the doors I wanted. I learned to trust the doors that do appear and to understand that they appear for a reason. I learned to have patience that a door will open when another closes. And that it's not the end of the world when things don't go as we want. I learned never to give up and never to feel sorry for myself. Even now, at age 68, after a stroke, I don't feel sorry for myself. I feel blessed for the opportunities I've had in life.

I'd say my experience of dying helped me to believe in myself when no one else did. It helped me stay motivated to always do my best in whatever situation I was in. And it taught me, too, that no authority is greater than God. That I can't let people tell me what my limitations are, because God's plan for me is different. And that's the plan I had to follow and not allow myself to get sidetracked feeling sorry for myself or allowing others to set my limitations. If I had allowed other people to set my limitations for me, I wouldn't have accomplished what I did in my life.

I do believe that things happen for a reason, that things come together and fall into place to give us what we need at that time in our lives. It's hard to understand these things as they happen, but looking back at my life I can see that specific events occurred to lead me down a path I believe I was meant to follow. It's just a matter of staying open to the idea that there's a reason why things happen as they do, even if we can't understand what that reason is at the time.

Exercise 1: Exploring Our Beliefs About Spirituality

The idea that we are all part of a grand plan—and that our lives have purpose—is a belief that is part of many religious and philosophical doctrines. The faith we have in such views often influences whether we interpret our life occurrences as senseless events or as opportunities to grow spiritually. When things are going well, we generally do not question the meaning of our lives. It is only when adversity befalls us that we begin to ponder the questions "Why?" and "For what purpose?" In your journal, record the following:

❧ Describe your beliefs about spirituality and the meaning of life. Ask yourself where you learned these beliefs. Have your present beliefs been shaped by childhood religious education or your parents' convictions? Have you rethought your views as a result of exposure to other religions and philosophies?

❧ In previous chapters you began to articulate your beliefs about illness or disability. Do your assumptions reflect the religious or spiritual beliefs you were raised with? Have you rethought your views based on later exposure to other religions and philosophies?

❧ What meaning does illness or disability have in the greater scheme of life, according to the spiritual beliefs you hold? Are they a random occurrence resulting from genetic anomalies or environmental pollutants? A test of faith?

❧ The notion of a just world involves the idea that we sow what we reap—that is, that people receive what they deserve based on their adherence to proper conduct. Is illness or disability incongruent with your belief in a just world? To what degree do you believe in the concept of a just world and the assumption that those who are moral should not experience suffering?

❧ Examine whether you hold resentment because you became ill despite your effort to live ethically, while others—who may have lived less virtuously—remain in good health. Do you find yourself asking questions such as "Why did this happen to me?" If so, try to move beyond this unanswerable question and instead ask yourself "What possible purpose could this illness or disability have in my life?"

🖋 Can you identify anything positive that you have learned from your experience thus far? Remember, we often cannot understand the value of certain life experiences—particularly those that cause great distress—until much later in our lives, when their meaning becomes apparent and we can appreciate what have we gained from that trauma.

Exercise 2: Identifying the Lessons of Our Spiritual Journey

Many religions and spiritual philosophies contend that all of our life events occur with meaningful intention. Moreover, some theologies suggest that we came into this human existence with our own life plan, replete with lessons designed to help us grow. The joy and misfortune that we experience occur with a purpose: to offer the understanding we are meant to acquire through human existence.

Imagine that a loving teacher has entered your life to help you understand the lessons of your life journey. Envision that you and your teacher embark on a review of the major events in your life—those both satisfying and distressful—and that during this review your teacher helps you better understand why a particular event occurred, how this experience encouraged your growth, and what hidden purpose it served in your life and in the lives of your loved ones. Record the following in your journal:

🖋 Begin with the major life events that happened in your childhood, and identify for your teacher what each event taught you. Proceed chronologically through the major events of your lifetime. Try to envision yourself as you experienced the event while you and your teacher observe from a distance. In this experience your teacher guides you toward the understanding that the adversity you endured was not meant as a form of punishment but rather as a learning opportunity that you could not comprehend at the time. Your teacher also helps you understand that the mistakes you made were part of your learning process rather than reason for you to inflict present self-torment.

᪽ Now advance to your present life. Ask if your teacher can help you better understand why you are experiencing illness or disability and how this circumstance is aiding your spiritual growth. Is illness or disability urging you to become more compassionate with yourself and others? Is it teaching you humility and the ability to accept help? Is it fostering gratitude for each day? Is it impelling you to reconsider that which is truly meaningful in your life? Are you learning to be more accepting and forgiving of yourself and others? Are you being urged to slow down and make lifestyle changes that could enhance your quality of life (and the lives of your loved ones)? Remember to thank your teacher for compassionately sharing these insights with you.

When you review your overall life lessons as they are listed chronologically in your journal, can you see any repeated themes or life lessons? Have multiple situations offered you the continued opportunity to learn a specific lesson? Often one life lesson requires several years to master, and several situations may be involved in teaching it. When viewing our life lessons as a list, it frequently becomes apparent that we needed to learn only a few simple lessons that continually emerge in differing guises throughout our life's journey.

Are you able to draw any connections between past lessons and those you have confronted through your experience of illness or disability? Often the lessons that we have been striving to master for most of our lives become clearer in the face of our illness or disability. Much as academic lessons become progressively difficult as we advance in school, life lessons tend to become more exacting with increasing age. Illness or disability is one of the most challenging of life's lessons.

It also is reassuring to observe that many other people have confronted the same life lessons we are confronting and that we are not alone in our need to acquire the skills we are meant to learn in this lifetime. If you are fortunate enough to participate in these exercises with a friend who is also experiencing illness or disability, compare your notes about life lessons. It is often heartening to observe the overlap between your own and your friend's lists. Such overlap is common because we frequently choose friends and favor loved ones who share similar learning needs; these relationships then reinforce our commitment to maintain the course on which we have embarked. Overlap of life lessons also is common because human existence provides opportunities to practice a set of lessons that are unique to the universal conditions of human life. People of the same generation may find that they share similar life lessons that differ from generations before or after. However, despite generational differences, a common universality exists for the types of lessons most often required in human existence.

Consider how the relationships in your lifetime have fostered your life lessons. People come and go throughout the ongoing seasons of our lifetimes, sharing our path for a while and then leaving, as though a chapter of a book has closed. We frequently discover that many of the people who played significant roles in one season are nowhere to be found—for one reason or another—in other seasons. Others remain as constant companions, sometimes playing the role of friend, at other times that of the challenger. The people who have entered our lives may have been significant to us or not, yet they all helped us to better learn the lessons on our life path. In a reciprocal way, we also helped them better acquire their own lessons.

Sometimes the relationships we have with others are hurtful, yet these relationships, too, have fostered our life lessons. Often our most meaningful lessons are learned through pain and loss. Think back to each of the major life seasons you plotted on the timeline of your life in Chapter 1, and identify the relationships that were significant at that time. Looking back, can you better understand how specific relationships helped you continue on your life path? Also, recall the relationships that did not seem significant at the time but that turned out to offer something important that was unfathomable in the moment.

Some theologians and philosophers believe that the full meaning of our lives remains hidden until the completion of this existence—that it is only then that we can fully comprehend the entire meaning underlying our life events and the connections between those occurrences and our life plan. Many people who prosper in the achievement of their life goals despite illness or disability echo this sentiment—that they had to surrender the need to understand why their illness or disability occurred and instead focus on learning how to make their lives livable in the present moment.

If you find that you have difficulty accepting your illness or disability and understanding why it has occurred, practice the exercises in Chapter 5 to maintain your attention in the present moment. Identify two activities you can participate in today to bring meaning to your life in the present. Select simple activities that can be easily carried out, such as telephoning a close friend or preparing a favorite meal. When your mind wanders to questions like "Why?" and "For what purpose?" catch these questions using mindfulness training.

Try replacing them with questions that instead ask "What will I do today to infuse meaning into my life?" and "How can I use what I've learned to help another person today?"

Exercise 3: Pondering the Idea That the Journey We Receive Is the One That We Need

Some believe that the life path on which we find ourselves is the one that we were meant to travel because it best matches our specific growth needs. Just as our journey would not be suitable for someone else, the life path of others—no matter how apparently favorable—would not best support our own development. This belief implies the broader idea that the universe operates to ensure that we receive what we need, rather than what we want, and that life is arranged in such a way that events fall into place under the guidance of a benevolent universe that respects our best interests, even if we cannot perceive this in moments of distress.

Sometimes we are able to gain glimpses of this process in everyday happenings. Coincidences occur in which needed events, no matter how trivial, fall into our laps or unfold in unexpected ways. Ellen, one of the interviewees for this book, experienced such a coincidence. She missed an appointment with a renowned doctor because she had incorrectly scheduled it in her calendar. Having waited for this appointment for a month, she berated herself for her carelessness and missed opportunity. She had canceled work to attend this appointment and spent the remainder of the day at home obliviously watching television as she ruminated "I can't believe I missed the appointment—I'm so thoughtless. I could have begun treatment that could be improving my health. Now I have to wait another three weeks. What a lost opportunity." As Ellen continued to berate herself, she became aware that a news segment had appeared on CNN about the very illness she had been diagnosed as having. The segment described an alternative treatment that researchers were beginning to find effective.

Ellen pursued this treatment and found it to be helpful where other treatments had failed. It was a year later that she realized that, by missing her appointment, she was able to be home at the precise time when the news segment aired—a seeming coincidence that benefited her health in the long run. When such coincidences happen, we often marvel at them and then forget them, interpreting their meaning as random events that occur with luck rather than as indicative of a universe that seeks to provide for us.

Can you recall seeming coincidences in your own life that ultimately benefited you or offered just what you needed? Have you ever followed a strong inner urge to engage in (or avoid) some activity and realized that your life would have been different had you not paid attention to such guidance? Paying greater attention to such apparent coincidences—for example, by maintaining an ongoing record of them—will enhance your ability to acknowledge such happenings. Maintaining a record of coincidences that benefited you also will reinforce your belief that events occur with meaningful intent.

When misfortune occurs, we must grieve and fully feel our emotions. But we can lessen our grief by remembering that adversity may herald something positive that we will understand only at a later time. Recognizing this possibility in the face of crisis often determines whether we feel victimized by our experiences or whether we can feel a sense of gratitude for the opportunities we have been offered, even if we cannot fully comprehend those opportunities in the moment. The next time you experience a disturbing event, feel your sorrow and distress but then practice considering the idea that something positive may eventually emerge from this situation that you cannot foresee. You do not need to understand how good may come from your suffering. Simply practice consciously holding the idea that something positive may eventually emerge. Practice until this thought becomes a habitual response whenever you experience adversity.

Exercise 4: Recognizing Our Identification With Our Body vs. Our Spirit

The experience of physical illness or disability often facilitates overidentification with our bodies. After all, with both we often strive to regain and preserve the health of our bodies against a physical process that has gone awry. Such focused concentration may cause us to lose sight of the idea that we are more than a physical body and that we may be allowing our illness or disability to adversely affect our spirit. Some describe the spirit as the life force that propels our motivation to press forward despite whatever tragedy we may endure. Some suggest that our spirit existed before human life and will continue to do so after our body has passed away. (See "Further Reading" for resources on Taoism, Buddhism, and mythology and the lessons of human life; see also Chopra and Ferrini.) It is said that our spirit uses the form of the physical body to experience human existence and the lessons we established for our growth rather than the other way around. When our lives become too focused on the preservation of the body at the expense of nurturing the spirit, life loses quality and meaning. Record your thoughts on the following in your journal:

 Examine whether you fear the eventual death of your body. Do not berate yourself for feeling fear, as this is a normal emotion that results from our attachment to the body—and attachment to the body also is natural after years of living with it. However, our fears of bodily death may be driving our efforts to heal the body at the expense of the spirit.

Ask yourself if you have become consumed with healing your body and have neglected to nourish your spirit. If you feel unhappy or disappointed much of the time, the answer to this question is probably yes. The Dalai Lama tells us that seeking to comfort or preserve the body will not bring happiness. (See "Further Reading" for writings of the Dalai Lama.) Rather, engaging in three simple activities that lighten our hearts is a better way to bring joy to our daily existence: (1) demonstrating compassion and love to others, (2) expressing our unique talents and abilities and thus sharing our gift with the larger world, and (3) trusting the belief that a benevolent universe will provide what we need to foster our spiritual growth.

Examine the degree to which these activities are present in your life. Often we may have excelled or overcompensated in one of the activities and have neglected the others. Identify one simple way that you can bring each activity into your daily existence. Performing these activities helps us remember our spiritual nature—that we are more than simply a body. They also enable us to extend this remembrance to others—to recall that others are spiritual beings, too.

NINE

FINDING THE GIFT
IN OUR EXPERIENCE
AND LISTENING TO THE
MESSAGES OF ILLNESS

There is a Buddhist saying that all crisis presents opportunity. (See "Further Reading" for resources on Buddhism.) One unique characteristic of the people who transformed their lives through illness or disability was their ability to find the gift—to understand and acknowledge the positive—that has come from their experience. Some spoke of the gift as an ability to better appreciate life instead of dwelling on the negative. Others expressed that the gift was their realization that they had to begin taking better care of themselves and the recognition that they are indeed worthy enough to treat themselves with compassion. Sometimes the gift came as a call to change aspects of their lifestyles—work, relationships, places of residence—to enhance the meaning and satisfaction of their lives. Many stated that the gift took the form of a deepening of their most meaningful relationships. But no matter how they described the gift, these people could pinpoint one or more positive events that occurred as a result of their illness or disability, that enriched their lives, and that likely would not have occurred—they believed—without their experience of crisis.

The Gift That Amy Found Through Illness

At 40, Amy had already become the senior copy editor of a national magazine based in New York City. In the winter after she was promoted to this position, Amy contracted a severe case of the flu that lingered through the following spring. After several more months of the same symptoms, she went to see her doctor who, after many tests, made a diagnosis of chronic fatigue syndrome, a condition believed to be caused by a viral infection (such as Epstein–Barr) that leaves people with low-grade fever, a sore throat, enlarged lymph nodes, muscle weakness, painful joints, headaches, and extreme exhaustion after participation in normal daily activities. Chronic fatigue syndrome also can be accompanied by sleep disturbances, decreased concentration, and depression—all of which Amy experienced.

THE YEAR BEFORE I WAS DIAGNOSED with chronic fatigue syndrome, I had just been promoted to the position of senior copy editor of the magazine I worked for. I had always worked hard and put in 60-hour weeks, but the responsibilities of this new job were even more demanding. Now I'd say I was averaging between 60- and 80-hour weeks. It was nothing for me to get to work at 7:30 in the morning and not leave until 10:00 at night. If we had an important story to cover, I often worked on the weekends. I didn't have time to think about how unbalanced my life had become because I was so busy trying to be successful at work. That winter was a bad flu season. It seemed as though every time I turned on the TV, I saw another newscast about flu epidemics and people dying from the flu.

I remember that the week between Christmas and New Year's was a quiet time that year. We had already completed the next issue of the magazine for the new year, and I was making plans to go on vacation in the Caribbean—I just wanted to get away from the coldness and gray of the city and be in a warm, sunny place. The morning that I was supposed to catch my plane, I woke up with a bad sore throat and intense body aches. And I knew that this was probably the flu, even though I had gotten a flu shot several months before. They said that the flu shots weren't hitting the strains that actually came around that year. I thought about getting up and dressed, but as I sat upright to get out of bed my head just spun and I got very dizzy and nauseous, and I knew that there was no way that I was traveling anywhere.

The next few days are all a blur. I was very sick—so sick that I couldn't get out of bed, I was vomiting and had diarrhea, and my lungs and sinuses had become very congested. My muscles were so sore that I was in constant pain. I couldn't even take any over-the-counter drugs because I couldn't keep anything down. And this went on for about 12 days. When the worst of the flu was over, I could get out of bed, but I had no strength. It took all my energy just to walk from the bedroom to my bathroom—and I have a small one-bedroom apartment. But I finally put myself in a cab and went back to work. For about a month I walked around with my nose constantly running and a sore throat that wouldn't go away. But everyone was sick, so I didn't seem out of place.

What concerned me most was how tired I was all the time. I mean, I was just really fatigued. By the time I'd get dressed in the morning and take the subway to work, I was ready to take a nap. I'd get to work and need an hour to get my energy back before I could concentrate on anything. I spent a lot of time flipping through papers, looking like I was busy, when I really had no idea what was going on—it was like being in a fog. And there was no way that I could put in the hours that I used to, so I made a lot of excuses about needing to leave early. If I would get home by 5:00 p.m. I'd collapse on the bed, often without eating anything, and then sleep through the night until the alarm went off the next morning. But I was never refreshed. No matter how much sleep I got, I was always in a state of extreme fatigue.

After walking around like this for four months, I decided that this wasn't normal and went to the doctor. I expected that either I had some rare incurable disease or she'd give me a drug that would knock this thing right out. Boy, was I wrong. Test after test revealed nothing, and I started thinking that this was all in my head—that maybe work had just gotten to me. And the doctor finally said that she thought I had chronic fatigue syndrome and that I could be walking around with this condition for who knows how long.

Over the next year I tried to maintain the lifestyle I had, but the pace of it got ridiculous—I just couldn't keep it up. So I had to make some pretty significant changes in my life. I went back to freelance writing because I could work at my own pace and set my own hours. I changed my entire diet. Before, I barely had time to eat. I'd grab a bagel for breakfast and eat lunch and dinner whenever I found time in the day. Most days I skipped either lunch or dinner. And whatever meal I could fit in was usually food from a street vendor; it wasn't exactly the most healthy way to eat. The rest was all candy bars and donuts, whatever stuff was in the office that day. Now I make sure that I eat three meals a day and get adequate supplies of protein and calcium, which I never did before. And of course, I'm now downing vitamin and mineral supplements like you can't believe. I also make sure that I get between seven and eight hours of sleep every night. No matter what deadline I'm under, I always make sure that I'm in bed by 11:00. Before this all happened, it wasn't at all uncommon for me to pull all-nighters to get an issue out. So I guess the chronic fatigue syndrome really forced me to make some very positive changes in my lifestyle.

Some days I'm fine. I wake up and feel that I have energy and can get work done. Other days—especially if I've pushed myself too much in the days before—I just want to sleep. It's all I can do to go to the grocery store to buy bread and milk. And that's the extent of my day. If I feel I'm getting a cold, I have to be extremely careful because a simple common cold, for me, could exacerbate the chronic fatigue and leave me incapacitated for several weeks.

If I had to assess how all of this has changed me, the first thing I'd say is that the illness has made me slow down. I was really rushing through life at a very fast pace. And my life had become all work and nothing else. Being forced to slow down because of illness—and some days not being able to do much of anything at all—has enabled me to become aware of so many other things that I never paid attention to. Now I value the time I have to write. I'm much more appreciative of the opportunity to have work that I enjoy and that I can accomplish on my own schedule. And I'm thankful for the ability to have a more balanced life—to be able to sit down at a table and eat a normal dinner, instead of gulping it down as an afterthought because a deadline is pressing. That's probably one of the best things to come out of this illness: that it made me change my lifestyle in healthy ways.

The other thing is that it provided the chance for me to resolve some issues I had with my mother and sister; it helped us all become closer. I was always very independent; I've never liked needing to ask for help. But an exacerbation of the chronic fatigue can be incapacitating—it can make me so sick that getting out of bed and getting dressed can be exhausting, cooking a meal and cleaning up afterward can be too tiring, and going to the store to buy a bag of groceries can be too much. It's a very regressive feeling to be an independent adult and need help for very basic daily activities. And it made me examine why I had so much trouble asking for help when I clearly needed it.

My mother was a single mom who raised me and my younger sister, and growing up I always felt that I was somewhat of a burden to my mom. She and my sister always had a better relationship, and I resented my sister for this. So by the time I was 18, I had moved out of my mother's house and went to school and worked in the city. And I really didn't want to be dependent on her or anybody. That's another thing that this illness has taught me: that sometimes in life you need to ask for help; you need to have someone to depend on. And I had to learn to ask for help because I was never any good at it. It's only now, after living with this illness for several years, that I realize this was all about my fear of rejection. I guess because I felt like a burden to my mother as a child, I also felt that I wasn't worth being cared for. And as an adult, when I needed her help, I was afraid that she'd reject me.

It was the same thing with my sister. She's been married and living in the suburbs for the past several years, and we really hadn't spoken much. We never developed an adult relationship as siblings. But because of my illness, we've become much closer. There were times when I have been very sick that she's taken me to her home and cared for me. If it wasn't for this illness, I'm sure that we'd never have gotten closer. I could have spent the rest of my life feeling distant from her and not knowing how much she loves me. I'm very thankful for this opportunity.

It's been the same with my mother. She's stayed with me in my apartment many times when I needed help. During these times she's taken care of me as though I were a child again—cooking for me, helping me bathe, helping me dress. And I know now how much she loves me as well. I'm not sure that I would have had the chance to experience this if I didn't get sick. It's ironic that a chronic health condition has helped me heal my relationship with my mother and sister. I think that's probably been the gift that has come out of this experience.

Exercise 1: Listening to the Message

Some people believe that illness or disability, like any major life event, brings a message with its appearance in our lives. Sometimes that message alerts us that something is amiss and urges us to make changes for the better. It is our responsibility, however, to hear and interpret the messages that illness or disability may hold for us.

Recognizing the Message to Slow the Pace of Life

For many people, illness or disability may indicate a need to slow the pace of their lifestyles. Often situations in which inactivity is forced on us offer a greater opportunity to turn inward and reflect on our lives, and the message of illness or disability is to urge us to slow down.

Like Amy, my own life had become very unbalanced and too fast paced. Before the car accident, in which I sustained cervical nerve impingement and chronic pain throughout my neck and back, I was often present at my job from 7:00 a.m. to 5:00 p.m. each weekday. I spent two more hours a day commuting from my home to the city and back.

After dinner, I would commonly exercise for an hour each night, go to sleep exhausted, wake up by 5:00 a.m. the next day, and repeat the cycle all over again. On the weekends I typically worked eight-hour days, thereby eliminating almost all the time I had for rest and leisure. Although I believed that I was physically caring for my body by maintaining a healthy diet and exercising, I was instead running my body into a state of depletion and exhaustion. The car accident I experienced forced me to stop working for a month. When I could return to work, I found that I could sustain neither the hours I was accustomed to nor the commute. I was no longer able to sit for hours at a computer; instead, I was forced to take frequent breaks and rest periods, and the pain was so debilitating that I could not work at my former rate.

This situation caused me to question whether I truly wanted to maintain the job and lifestyle I had lived with for so many years. I unequivocally believe that the accident was a message to slow down and exchange the frenzied lifestyle I had created for one that supported greater time for rest, leisure, and balanced activity. Illness compelled me to make these positive lifestyle changes. I doubt that I would have created such changes on my own, because I had lived this way for so many years that I was accustomed to it and was resistant to change—despite how exhausted and dissatisfied I had become. In this sense, illness was a gift, as it helped me reconfigure a lifestyle that was healthier and more personally satisfying. Illness, too, was an alarm, not simply indicating that conditions were amiss in my physical body but also that conditions in my life as a whole had injured my emotional health.

Consider the pace of your life. Does it feel comfortable? Or do you feel that you never have enough time? Are you spending time participating in the activities you truly desire? Or do activities feel more like never-ending chores that are done out of necessity? Is illness or disability a sign to slow down or to make changes in the way you are organizing your day?

❧ *Recognizing the Message That We Deserve to Ask for What We Need*

Sometimes illness or disability emerges in our life to help us learn to become better advocates for ourselves, to offer us an opportunity to learn to ask for what we want or need. This is especially true for people who must learn to advocate for their medical needs in a health care system that attempts to cut costs at the expense of quality and that considers the patient to be a passive recipient of services performed by authorities. Fighting insurance companies for needed services—particularly when illness or disability has depleted our energy—is a powerful tool through which to learn self-advocacy.

However, learning to advocate for ourselves also can involve becoming more proficient at understanding our emotional needs and expressing those needs to loved ones. We may still unconsciously embrace beliefs that we are not worthy enough to request that our needs be met. This may be true particularly if we grew up in an environment in which our needs were not considered important by our caretakers. Illness or disability may act as a message that we need to question this belief and recognize that we deserve to ask for what we need. Both also teach that our needs are no more or less important than anyone else's.

Conversely, illness or disability can be the great humbler and equalizer. If we are not accustomed to asking for or accepting help from others out of pride or an extreme need for independence, illness or disability teaches that we are not superior to others—that we all share the same human experience, that asking for and accepting help is part of being human, and that no one is so self-sufficient that they do not need assistance at one time or another. Illness or disability may teach us how to accept help from others if we have never been accustomed to asking for and receiving assistance.

Think back to whether your needs were met in childhood. Did your parents (or caretakers) convey that your needs were important? Or did you receive the message that your needs created problems? Did you learn to suppress your needs? Were you given the message—directly or indirectly—that you should learn to take care of your needs alone?

Consider whether it is difficult for you to advocate for your medical needs in the present. How well you are able to advocate for your own needs may be directly related to whether your needs were addressed or valued in childhood. Consider how easily you are able to ask your loved ones for help when needed. Do you often refrain from asking for assistance because you feel that you may be bothering others who have their own problems? Do you fear that, by asking for help, you will become a burden to your loved ones?

When we need assistance and do not ask for it, two things happen: (1) We miss the opportunity to receive what we need, and (2) we deny others the opportunity to build intimacy with us by offering their help. If you experience difficulty expressing your needs to others, identify one need that is not burdensome, and practice how you might communicate this need to a loved one. Put into words the fact that you feel uncomfortable making the request but that the assistance you are seeking would be of great benefit to you. Be sure to communicate your request without using guilt to influence the other to offer assistance.

☙ Recognizing the Message to Take Better Care of Ourselves

Illness or disability also can warn us that we need to take better care of ourselves. Many people who overcome addictions state that hitting rock bottom saved their lives because it made them understand—when nothing else could—that if they did not change their behaviors, they would die. I have heard the same sentiments from young people whose risk-taking behaviors (commonly driving while intoxicated) have contributed to severe head injuries that left them with paralysis and cognitive deficits. To my great initial surprise, many of these young adults expressed appreciation for their accidents, because they recognized that the accident and rehabilitation gave them another chance to live. I remember the words of 23-year-old John, whose car accident left him in a wheelchair and requiring assistance for every activity of daily living: "The way I was going, I would have been dead in a year's time. The stuff I was into, the crazy things I did while I was high. I know that I got a second chance to live because of my accident. And I'm grateful for it."

Sometimes illness or disability signals that we need to change the way we care for ourselves in more subtle ways—the foods we eat to nourish our health, the amount of exercise we undertake, how meticulously we comply with our medication requirements, how much rest we allow our bodies to heal. Identify whether your illness or disability may carry a message to make changes in the ways you take care of yourself. Because change is always difficult, even when desired, begin by selecting two modest changes you wish to make that would help you better care for yourself. Perhaps you want to ensure that you get sufficient restorative sleep to allow your body time to heal by establishing set times to sleep and wake. Try going to bed and waking at the same times every day and night for one week. Or perhaps you would like to eat more healthfully. Try to eat a single healthy meal per day for one week, and gradually incorporate healthier foods into every meal. Record your attempts in your journal, and monitor your progress over the next weeks.

Remember that change takes time and is characterized by an uneven course of gains and setbacks. Do not berate yourself for the setbacks; rather, understand that they are a normal part of the change process and should be expected.

✒ Recognizing the Message to Spend Our Time in Meaningful Ways

Illness or disability also may be a message that we need to spend more time participating in meaningful activities. When we assess how we spend the hours of each day and week, we commonly find that much of our time is spent in activities that are emotionally draining, unsatisfying, mentally unstimulating, or burdensome. Illness or disability—and a sense of metered time—often compels us to begin participating in activities that we desire but have continually delayed. Many people experiencing illness or disability engage in long-desired travel, complete their education, or spend more time with family and friends.

Examine whether your illness or disability carries a message to begin engaging in activities that bring meaning to your life. If you feel that too many of your hours are wasted on activity that you neither enjoy nor find satisfying, this is a clear sign to change how you spend your time. We will always have to participate in daily activity that is unpleasant but necessary, such as household chores. But we can reorganize our time used for such necessities to increase our time available for desired activities. For example, if you dislike cooking, you may be able to decrease meal preparation time by purchasing precooked or freshly prepared food items that are ready to serve and require little cleanup. It may be necessary to limit activity that encroaches on time you would rather spend otherwise, such as refraining from answering the telephone for a designated period of each day or grocery shopping when crowds and lines are at a minimum.

Next, focus on how you would like to spend more of your time—identify the activities you wish to engage in, and consider whether you could incorporate these daily, weekly, or monthly. Then schedule a designated time into your day (or week or month) when you can participate in such pursuits. Begin with one modest activity that is relatively easy to fit into your current lifestyle, for example, making time to read for 15 minutes before bed. Tell your family members that you are seeking to incorporate a specific activity into your day, and request their support. It is beneficial to maintain a record of your participation in desired activities; note whether they actually took place and, if not, what prevented their occurrence. Such a record will help you understand how to better plan your time to ensure that desired activities will indeed occur.

Do not feel disappointed if your desired activities do not always occur; in fact, you should expect that they will not occur a certain percentage of time. However, that percentage should not exceed 50%. If the activities you desire most are not happening at least 50% of the time, you may need to reorganize your schedule to better support your participation in these activities.

Simplifying our lives is another way to reclaim lost time and restore sanity to a chaotic lifestyle. Watch what responsibilities you assume. Be cautious not to assume responsibilities that belong to others or that others can carry out. Do not succumb to the temptation of assuming responsibility simply because you are the most competent person to complete certain tasks or because others expect you to. Choose your commitments wisely and with realistic consideration of the amount of energy and time you have. Select your medical treatment with the same consideration. Sometimes treatment is so involved and time-consuming that we have no energy left for anything else that could enhance the quality of our lives; we may extend the length of our lives by some degree, but at the cost of quality.

◟ *Recognizing the Message to Appreciate What We Have in the Present*

Illness or disability may help awaken our appreciation for the present moment and the gifts we have been given in our lives thus far. We often do not value the abundance we have been offered, instead focusing on our disappointment and dissatisfaction with the way our expectations have not been fulfilled. Illness or disability, and the prospect of losing our way of life as we know it, can instill gratitude for the gifts we have trivialized or overlooked.

In Chapter 5 you began to engage in exercises that helped you understand and appreciate the gifts in your everyday life. Has your illness or disability enabled you to experience greater conscious appreciation for a loved one's companionship? For the ability to enjoy a favorite meal, cherished music, or the unconditional love with which your pet greets you? Has your illness or disability encouraged your thankfulness for another day to live? Both can often teach us to appreciate and value the mundane events of life that we tend to depreciate. The ability to value the mundane is one of the most significant gifts, because it allows us to remain focused in the present moment and to savor that time. Worrying about the future or regretting the past falls by the wayside as we recognize that the present moment is immeasurably valuable. Our ability to acknowledge our gratitude for the present moment—and our desire not to waste the time we have available—becomes heightened.

◟ *Recognizing the Message to Heal Broken Relationships*

Illness or disability also may be a message that we need to mend relationships severed by conflict. Illness or disability—

and the prospect of an end to this life—often casts conflict in a different perspective. Both allow us to shift our perspective from the thick of the trees (and the dramas they represent) to the forest from a distance, enabling us to see the larger picture. We come to recognize that the forest is made up of many interrelated parts and that every being—even the smallest insect—is important to the forest's survival as a whole.

In our own lives we benefit by acknowledging the interrelationships we have with others and the importance of such dependence in fostering our survival in this world. Illness or disability encourages us to mend relationships with people about whom we have felt resentment, anger, and judgment. These feelings only separate us from greater intimacy and companionship. Often events that caused outrage and turmoil seem trivial in the face of illness and mortality. When we recognize that such a perspective is indeed a gift, we begin to understand that illness or disability is a path to greater tolerance and acceptance and that, without tolerance and acceptance, we cannot receive the greater gift of inner peace.

In Chapter 3 you began to examine whether forgiveness was needed in any of your relationships. Ask yourself again if you have unhealed relationships that may be disturbing your peace of mind. Review the exercises in Chapter 3 to mend relationships in which forgiveness is required. Remember that, when we offer love and forgiveness to others, we offer it to ourselves—we remove a burden that weighs heavily on our hearts and minds. Conversely, when we withhold love and forgiveness from others, we diminish our opportunity to experience these directly, and the burden of conflict remains heavy on our spirit.

Recognizing the Message to Heal Negative Emotions

Illness or disability often prompts inner reflection and contemplation of life as a whole. Because people experiencing illness or disability are commonly forced to spend a great deal of time alone with their thoughts, illness or disability frequently affords them the opportunity to pay closer attention to their emotions. Emotions that have remained unconscious are commonly brought to light for greater examination. And because both tend to exacerbate fear, sadness, anger, and guilt, we are offered a unique opportunity to explore and resolve emotions we may otherwise ignore or deny. In this way illness or disability can be cleansing, as both force us to deal with emotions that we typically disregard and neglect. Without such conscious examination, repressed emotions commonly wreak havoc in our lives, as they tend to be expressed unconsciously through destructive words and behaviors.

In Chapter 6 you began to explore your emotions of fear, sadness, anger, and guilt to acknowledge, accept, and release these feelings. In this chapter, we recognize the gift we have been given through the opportunity to examine and release the negative emotions that might otherwise have remained unconscious if illness or disability had not forced them into our conscious awareness. Review the exercises in Chapter 6 to determine if you still hold negative emotions requiring further healing and release.

Recognizing the messages that illness or disability has brought into our life affords the unique opportunity to make positive lifestyle changes. Rather than viewing illness or disability as a taskmaster whose goal is punishment, we can appreciate illness or disability as a teacher who compassionately offers the guidance we need to make our lives more livable and to learn the lessons we require for this life path. When we hear the messages that both reveal, we have received a gift of communication offered with healing intention. Such messages are akin to signposts along the path of our life journey, meant to guide our decisions and actions toward our own best interests.

What major gifts brought to your life through illness or disability have you identified? What are the major messages you have received? Record these in your journal, and review them periodically to maintain your perspective on occasions when you feel that you are fighting an uphill battle.

Exercise 2: Acknowledging the Gift of Time That Illness or Disability Brings

Illness or disability also grants the gift of time in which to express love and gratitude to family members and to say goodbye if needed. One of the most unsettling experiences of human life occurs when people either fail to take advantage of occasions to communicate their love or never have the opportunity to do so because of a loved one's sudden and unexpected death. The chance to express love and parting sentiments sometimes marks the difference between a grieving experience that heals with time and one that leaves a hole in a loved one's life spirit. In this light, illness or disability does not deprive us of time; rather, it compassionately offers the opportunity to experience closure in our most cherished relationships—to say goodbye and to verbalize the love and gratitude that, if left unsaid, can haunt our loved ones' lives.

None of us will live forever, but death for most people is a distant possibility. Illness enhances our awareness of mortality. Such an awareness commonly compels us to use the time we have available in the present to communicate words of importance to our loved ones. Are there people in your life to whom you would like to communicate specific sentiments? Do you want to convey your love and gratitude for their presence in your life or your pride in their accomplishments?

Identify the people with whom you would like to share your emotions before the opportunity to do so is no longer available. Identify the sentiments you desire to communicate. Consider the medium through which you would like to convey your emotions—are you skillful at finding just the right words to express your feelings in the moment? Or do you feel more comfortable expressing your thoughts in writing? Some people use audio- and videotapes to record their messages to loved ones so that such moments can be preserved.

Regardless of the medium you choose to express yourself, do not wait until you are no longer here to share your feelings. Communicating your emotions in the present does three things: (1) It allows both you and your loved ones to reach greater intimacy in the present, (2) it affords you and your loved ones the opportunity for closure if death is near, and (3) it offers your loved ones a chance to respond to your communication and share their own feelings. Waiting until after your death to disclose communications of love— through videotapes or writing—will not afford the same opportunity for closure as doing so in the present.

Sometimes, however, our loved ones do not wish to engage in final partings. If this is the case, try to compassionately convey to your loved ones that you want to take advantage of the present time that your illness or disability has afforded to share your feelings with them. Express that you do not want to miss this opportunity and that such time is a gift for both of you. If a loved one is strongly resistant, it may be best to use the medium of writing or taping your communication for your loved one to experience at a later time.

Exercise 3: Using the Gift of Life-Altering Purpose

Occasionally, illness or disability either offers a sense of purpose in our lives or alters the purpose we had been familiar with. Bill was a 25-year-old investment banker employed by a top-10 brokerage company. In 1995 he sustained a spinal cord injury and mild brain damage when his car was struck head on by a drunk driver. The accident caused paralysis of his legs and moderate memory deficits. By 1997, Bill had begun volunteering as a guest speaker and advocate for Mothers Against Drunk Driving and for the disability rights movement. He was averaging three public speaking occasions per month and was traveling both nationally and internationally. Bill stated that the accident changed both the direction of his life and his sense of life purpose.

Before my accident, everything was about making money and achieving material success. To be truthful, I really didn't think too much about anyone but myself. I didn't go out of my way to hurt anyone; it's just that other people were not on my mind—unless they could help me achieve my own goals. When I had my accident, I really thought that my life was over. I couldn't see past what I had lost. I wished that I had died that night. But during rehab I was introduced to another guy who had a similar accident and injury. He was lecturing at the local high schools and churches about drunk driving, and he got me involved in it. And it changed my life. I've been doing this for eight years now, and I'm truly a different person than I was before my accident. I can't even believe I'm the same guy.

Looking back, I'd have to say that the accident and my injury changed the way I think about the purpose of my life. I don't even think that I felt any purpose before then. But now I really believe that I was meant to help people understand how alcoholism can ruin your life. I feel—at least I hope—that my message is saving lives. I know I'm doing something of value that's helping people. And I feel really good about that. There's no comparison between the sense of purpose I feel in my life now and any that I might have felt before my accident. It's just night and day.

For most people, illness or disability will not reveal or transform a sense of life purpose in the dramatic way that Bill experienced. When illness or disability does recast the course of one's life purpose, such an experience is often a life-altering gift that can be understood only later. From your present vantage point, can you discern if your illness or disability has changed your sense of life purpose? How has the direction of your life path changed?

For most of us, illness or disability changes our life direction more subtly and over a greater period of time. We may be too close to our illness or disability to be able to understand how it has altered our life course and sense of meaning. If you could choose the specific ways your illness or disability altered your sense of purpose and life course, what would you choose? Imagine yourself two years from now. In what ways would you like your life to be different because of illness or disability? How will illness or disability have positively altered your life path and purpose? Record your thoughts in your journal so that you can periodically refer back to them—remember, all change begins as thought. How can you bring your thoughts into reality?

Identify two practical methods through which you can begin to set the course for positive change to occur in your life direction and sense of purpose. Each week for the next month, monitor whether you were able to work toward your desired goal. Even if you were able to only think about desired change, it is important to recognize that such thought lays the foundation for later action. Change is a difficult process that requires discipline, commitment to your goals, and patience. In six months, and then again in one year, refer back to the journal entry in which you described your desired changes in life direction and purpose. Acknowledge any effort made toward your goals. Do not devalue small progress or berate yourself if change did not happen. Remember, you have planted seeds that require a long time to mature. Although you may see little of the change you hoped for, progress may indeed be occurring in ways that you cannot understand from your present vantage point.

TEN

USING WHAT WE'VE LEARNED TO HELP OTHERS AND TO HEAL OURSELVES

In *The Hero With a Thousand Faces*, Joseph Campbell described a spiritual quest found in myths and folklore across human cultures. The hero, who symbolizes every human being, leaves the familiar and safe environment of his or her home and travels through the underworld, symbolizing a life-altering crisis that he or she must overcome as part of the journey. The hero emerges from this underworld to carry life wisdom back to the people at the home left behind to benefit humanity.

In almost every interview with the people who had transformed their lives through illness or disability, this same symbolic story appeared, along with the determination to use what they had learned through their pain and loss to help others similarly challenged. Perhaps this is one of the ways that humans across time and cultures attempt to make sense of a seemingly senseless illness or disability. Many of the people interviewed for this book stated that their ability to help others was the gift they found in their experience of crisis, and many expressed that giving something back was one of the most important keys to their own emotional healing and ability to find meaning in life.

Laura's Use of Her Experience to Help Others

Laura was an energetic and spirited 29-year-old speech pathologist who easily motivated her patients with her exuberance and compassion. At first glance, no one would ever believe that she had been in a severe car accident at age 5 that left her comatose for two months and caused significant brain damage and loss of speech.

I'VE ALWAYS FELT SEPARATE FROM what other people were experiencing in their lives. I lost my dad in the car accident, and so much of my identity as a child was tied up with his death. I grieved for him for years, and I couldn't let go because I thought if I did, I'd be letting go of my father. I'm 29 now, and it's only been recently that I've realized that I've been grieving all these years. I'm finally giving up that grief and trying to understand who I am as an adult.

But as a child, the accident set me apart from other children my age. First, I lost a lot of time in school because of the months I spent in the hospital. And then I had a lot of cognitive problems from my head injury, which are still with me today to some degree. My memory is not as good as it could be. Organizing a lot of details in my mind is harder than for most people. Sometimes I have a harder time understanding ideas or comprehending things.

Then, because he died in the car accident, I grew up without a father. And growing up, I think that I took on the identity of the little girl in the neighborhood who lost her father. It always seemed that my friends were doing things on the weekends with their dads, going places and stuff. Or it always seemed like there were too many father–daughter days at my school. I'm not sure there were—it was just the way I perceived it because I missed him so much. And I felt the lack of his presence in my life so acutely.

The other thing was that, because of the brain damage, I lost my speech for about a year. It took several years of speech therapy before I could speak clearly and audibly again. I remember what that was like as a little girl, not being able to talk. I wanted so much to be able to talk to my mother and to the other children in my neighborhood. It was very hurtful to me, and I felt very much like an outcast. So I tried 10 times harder at everything just to show people that I wasn't different, I wasn't slow. School wasn't easy for me; I guess because of the brain damage I always had trouble. But I was very determined to try my best and to succeed at my goals. No matter how many obstacles I faced, I always had faith in my ability to persevere.

When I was in high school, the guidance counselors told me that no college wanted me because my reading scores were so low and my grades weren't good enough. And I would say, "No, I can do it. I'm going to put my mind to it, and I *will* get into school." When things are hard, I always think, "God didn't let me die that day." All of the doctors thought that I was going to die. And then they said that if I lived, I'd never speak and I'd be paralyzed. And I can speak, and I'm not paralyzed. When things are hard, I always remember that the doctors were wrong about me. And this encourages my belief in myself—that I can go further and do more than what others believe I can do. I could have died in the accident, but I didn't. I really believe that there's meaning in why I'm here today.

When I got accepted into college—which they said I never would—I knew that I had to choose something that I enjoyed and that made sense to me about why I'm here and what I'm supposed to do with my life. I knew that I wanted to become a speech therapist, because this had personal meaning for me. Because of my own injury, I understood what the lack of speech can do to someone's life, and I knew that I wanted to help others in a way that I had been helped. I realize that not everyone who has experienced the injury I sustained has been able to recover as well as I have. I've been very lucky, and I feel that God has given me this chance, and I want to give back to others. So when I made the decision to become a speech therapist, it just seemed right—as though this is what I had to do; this is one of the reasons why I'm here. And from that day on, I didn't let anything stand in my way to reach this goal.

Now when I work, I often say to myself, "I know that I was meant to be here to help this person function again." I can understand all of their frustrations and fears because I've been there—I've been on the other side. I feel like I have to give back. After what I've been through, I feel that it's a gift from God to be able to speak, to be able to share with people what you're feeling, what you need, what you want. And because I understand what my patients are going through, I think it makes me a better therapist. I think that I have more patience and empathy for my patients, because I know first-hand what they're experiencing. And I think that it makes me try harder with my patients—particularly with patients whom other therapists have given up on. I don't believe there's any lost cause or any patient who's so far gone that we should give up on them. The doctors didn't think I'd make it or ever walk or speak again; they thought that I was a lost cause. And that taught me that there are no lost causes. I'll do whatever I can until God decides that it's that person's time.

I usually won't bring up my own experience with a patient unless they give up on themselves and stop trying to get better. When I'm with a patient who has lost hope, that's when I open up and share what happened to me. And when I do that, patients connect to me better and try harder. If they give up, they don't even know if they can potentially get better—they don't know the resources and strength they may have to rebuild their lives. I always say to them, "It's not the therapist who makes you better, it's you who makes you better."

Sometimes sharing my own story with patients gives them hope that if someone else can do it, they can do it too. And they usually do. Whenever I share my experience with a patient who has given up, they usually regain some ability to functionally speak again. And to be able to help people regain this function—it just makes me feel good. It makes me feel that I'm doing what I'm supposed to be doing with my life.

I also believe that I have a greater appreciation than other therapists for the hope that patients need to have. And I think that this came from my own experience of needing to have hope that tomorrow will not be worse, that tomorrow will be better. I remember trying to speak as a child, and nothing would come out. I know what that feels like, how frustrating it is. I know how my patients feel and how much they need to maintain their hope. So I'm always careful about what I say to patients to make sure that I'm instilling hope and not taking it away. People who have hope seem to be able to manage insurmountable challenges. People who give up really don't do as well. They become detached from their rehab and stop trying to help themselves.

And when I'm with my patients, I give 100% of my attention to them. I stop thinking about myself, and I'm fully with that patient, focusing totally on their needs. I forget myself. I forget whatever problems I may have. And this makes me feel good, and it's something that I try to take into other areas of my life. I try to listen deeply to my family and my friends when they talk to me. I try to let them know that I care about them. I try to reinforce the hope they have that they can achieve their own goals. And I try to be as compassionate with them as I can be because I understand what it's like to need compassion and not receive much of it.

I've found that the more I'm able to use my experience to help others, the more I feel healed from the trauma I went through. The more I know that I've helped another person because of what I went through, the less pain I feel about losing my father. Because I really feel that my dad is watching over me, helping me. I feel that he's with me in my daily life as I work with patients and just go about my day. It's like I have a new relationship with him now. I've come to believe that I had to go through the losses I experienced so that I could understand loss and help others go through it. And this belief has helped me heal the grief I've always walked around with for my dad. It's like the pain is finally beginning to lift after all these years.

Exercise 1: Recognizing the Difference Between Appropriate and Inappropriate Help

Extending help to others is commonly the one consistent and lasting method through which we can lift our spirits. Although material comforts and physical pleasures may alleviate our pain in the moment, that moment passes, and the gratification of materiality diminishes. The positive feelings that we derive from helping others have a profound effect on our inner well-being, in contrast to the more transient feelings produced by material pleasures. Helping others unshackles our focus on our own problems. This shift in attention from our concerns to another's brings our dilemmas into greater perspective. Through aiding others, we are able to create bonds, build intimacy, and feel connected to other people—which, in turn, enhances our own emotional health.

Helping others who experience authentic need, however, differs from inappropriately assuming responsibility for others' problems. Appropriate offerings of help neither drain our emotional resources nor oblige us to sacrifice our needs for those of others. The desire to assist others does not require that we never refuse another's request. Instead, we must balance protecting our own needs and limitations and providing help when we are able. In situations in which another's appeal for help is appropriate, no one's needs are sacrificed or subordinated—instead, the needs of all are respected equally. No one inappropriately surrenders his or her needs for others, and no one assumes responsibility that belongs to others.

Those who learned to assume a caretaker role in their families as children often continue to inappropriately assume caretaking in adulthood. They enter relationships in which they improperly assume another's responsibilities. Consider the following, and record your thoughts in your journal:

❦ Did you learn to be a caretaker in childhood? Were you the child who always took care of younger siblings? Did you help a parent or assume parenting roles because one or both parents were unavailable or unable to fulfill parental responsibilities? If you did learn caregiver behaviors in childhood, it is doubly important that you examine whether you know the difference between offering help appropriately and assuming responsibility that belongs to others.

🖉 Examine the types of relationships you have entered as an adult. Have you assumed a caretaking role in any of these relationships with other adults?

Helping others also does not mean that we impose our own will and expectations on them. Attempting to repair others in accordance with our assumptions about their need for help—particularly when the others do not agree that they require advice or remediation—does not constitute help. When we try to fix others who neither desire our help nor believe that they need assistance, we may do two things: (1) We may, inadvertently, convey the disrespectful message that they are not capable of helping themselves and that someone else knows what they need better than they do, and (2) we may confiscate their opportunity to learn to use their own resources to enhance their life circumstances. When we impose our own expectations and desires onto others, we begin to live their lives for them—we prevent them from traveling their own journey.

We have all attempted to change other people before we recognized that this is not only an impossibility but also disrespectful of another's rights to live in accordance with their inner guidance. Identify occasions when you attempted to impose your will (in an attempt to be helpful) on someone who did not desire your advice. Parents are often guilty of such actions with their children; spouses, too, commonly impose their will on each other, all in the guise of love and desire for another's best interest. Because we do not wish to see our loved ones make hurtful mistakes, we attempt to exert our control over their decisions and actions, often with unsatisfactory results.

When we attempt to control others, we take power from them, we convey that they are not capable of caring for themselves, and we prevent them from learning their own life lessons. Remember, the more we seek control, the more life slips out of our control. Consider these questions, and record your thoughts in your journal:

✺ On those occasions when you attempted to impose your helpfulness on someone who did not desire it, what happened? Was that person appreciative or resentful? Was conflict or harmony created in your relationship? Were you able to deepen the bonds and intimacy you hoped for?

✺ Do you feel compelled to offer your advice when others confide their concerns? Sometimes the most effective way to help is to listen deeply without offering suggestions. The next time someone shares a personal dilemma with you, do not rush to solve the situation. Instead, practice listening intently with your full attention. Listening deeply conveys your care and concern. Ask the person to articulate what he or she believes is the right thing to do. Often people need to rehearse their options verbally before selecting one path to follow. Encourage others to listen to their own gut feelings and inner voice. Allow them to make decisions with trust in their inner guidance; instill confidence in their ability to use that inner guidance to make the best decision. Remember, another's inner guidance emerges from a source that is far more capable of offering insight and advice than we are.

Exercise 2: Using What We Learn Through Illness or Disability to Help Others

When we review our lives from the perspective of age, we hope that we have positively contributed to the lives of others. Contributions that enhanced the welfare of others are often the achievements we are most proud of. Mythology and theology reflect the common theme that the experience of human life grants us the opportunity to help our fellow beings and that the crises we experience on our life journey occur with purpose—because it is through crisis that we learn our greatest lessons and are then asked to use our new knowledge to help others.

❧ In your journal, describe your personal story of the hero's journey with yourself in the role of the hero. What insight and knowledge have you gained from your journey—and your experience of crisis—that can assist others? How can you use your experience of illness or disability to enhance the lives of others?

The mentoring relationship is one of the most significant ways to extend help to another. People who successfully transcend traumatic events commonly reported that having a mentor who guided them through crisis was an important factor in their healing. Some became mentors to people recently receiving a similar diagnosis. In my work with people who have sustained traumatic brain injury, I have observed that connecting patients with a mentor who also had experienced brain injury and who was now living a life of quality often influenced whether patients would experience a positive rehabilitation. Many reported that their mentor served as a role model for the way they could rebuild their lives, particularly when they had lost hope of creating a viable post-injury life.

❧ Have you been fortunate to have a mentor who offered guidance throughout your experience of illness? If not, would you have benefited from knowing someone who could have shared information, assisted you in forming appropriate expectations, and helped you understand how to make life more livable with illness? Is mentoring an activity you would like to contribute to others?

Some find that initiating support groups—or facilitating ones already in existence—provides the opportunity to use their personal knowledge of illness to assist others. Several of the people interviewed for this book implemented or joined advocacy groups for people experiencing specific illnesses. These groups became a forum for sharing resources and emotional support with people who have similar health conditions. Many others made career changes that enabled them to use their experience of illness or disability to assist others daily.

We do not have to seek broad public forums, however, to feel that we are using our experience to make a positive difference in others' lives. Even people who do not have a great deal of energy or time can help others in their immediate environment—in their families and neighborhoods. Sometimes simply providing an opportunity for others to regain more of their own time, particularly during crisis, can be one of the most consequential ways to extend help. Offering to watch children while parents attend medical appointments or preparing a home-cooked meal for a family experiencing the illness or disability of a parent can be of great value. Frequently, the most meaningful ways to offer assistance are through ordinary mundane activities that are necessary for daily survival.

Imparting our wisdom from one generation to the next is another way to use our experience of adversity to help loved ones prevail through their own crises. Martha maintained a journal of the insights she learned from her illness and left it in her will to her children to help them survive their own trials. Her loving words and wisdom about life are recorded for posterity and continue to provide strength to her loved ones during periods of distress.

❧ Identify two ways that you can offer assistance to others in your environment during the next few weeks. Describe these experiences in your journal, and record the feelings you experienced in response to your offer of help.

Exercise 3: Identifying the Contributions for Which We Want to Be Remembered

If you are having trouble finding ways to transform your illness or disability experience into an opportunity to help others, consider what contributions you would like to be remembered for in your family or community. Would you like your family members or neighbors to remember you for the kind and reassuring words you spoke when others felt dejected? Would you like to be remembered for the way you readily welcomed people into your home? Or for the compassionate way you listened when someone approached you with a problem?

Again, it is not necessary to offer assistance on a grand scale to make a difference in someone's life. Frequently, our most meaningful contributions occur when we are able to convey that we care about others. We can achieve this through simple methods, like deeply listening, expressing feelings of love and acceptance, encouraging others to maintain effort during times of adversity, and expressing confidence in others' abilities and talents. People who overcome a great crisis or negative life conditions characteristically state that there was at least one person in their lives who demonstrated caring and concern, who listened, who encouraged them through difficulties, and who demonstrated belief in their abilities. If we can do this for one person, we will have positively contributed to someone's life more than we will ever know.

Remember, the seeds of all action begin as thought. Imagine the ways that you can contribute to others' lives. Then imagine how you can convert your thoughts into real-life behaviors. Often, just having the desire to help will bring opportunities directly to you. When such opportunities appear in your life, recognize that they are gifts that can help you transform your experience of illness or disability into a way to help others.

Exercise 4: Recognizing That What We Give to Others, We Also Give to Ourselves

There is an Eastern saying that what we give to others, we also give to ourselves. (See "Further Reading" for resources on Taoism and Buddhism.) Every act of kindness or compassion that we demonstrate to others is one that we also demonstrate to ourselves. Conversely, withholding love and assistance from others is akin to withholding these from ourselves.

Think back to a situation in which you helped another. Do you remember the positive feelings you experienced witnessing that person's gratitude for your assistance? Think back to a time when you expressed your love to someone who openly received it, and how good it felt (identify a non-romantic situation, as romantic love tends to distort our perceptions). Grandparents and dedicated teachers are familiar with the feelings obtained when we give of ourselves selflessly and without expectation to help another. When we help others without thought of return (and when we are not inappropriately assuming others' responsibilities), we tap into this phenomenon—we instantly feel the love and compassion we are bestowing.

It is said, too, that how we treat others is a reflection of whether we feel deserving of compassion, love, and kindness. (See "Further Reading" for resources on Taoism and Buddhism; see also Ferrini.) If we cannot treat others with compassion and kindness, it reflects that we truly do not know how to treat ourselves in this way. Often we learn how to help others by receiving help ourselves. We learn how to treat others with compassion and kindness by receiving the same treatment in our own life—by having someone who loves us enables us to feel what it is like to be treated benevolently and with consideration. Ask yourself if you know how it feels to be treated with gentleness and compassion.

If we have not had the experience of being treated with these qualities, however, it is not necessary to depend on the kindness of others to learn how to extend such compassion to ourselves. We can learn to treat ourselves with greater kindness by treating others in the same fashion. What we demonstrate to others will, in time, come to be reflected in our behaviors toward ourselves. Again, our ability to learn self-love is often directly connected to our ability to give love to our fellow human beings.

As noted before, often the most direct and powerful ways we can treat others compassionately and kindly are the most simple: offering a smile to express love and acceptance, verbalizing kind and reassuring words that lighten others' hearts, listening intently to another's concerns instead of rushing to offer advice or complaining about our own dilemmas, remembering special occasions, acknowledging someone's talent, and encouraging another's effort to reach personal goals. These are effective ways to make a difference in someone's day-to-day life. They do not require a great deal of time, energy, money, resources, or special effort. All they require is the genuine desire to treat others compassionately and thereby make a positive difference in someone's day.

Such acts can have a domino effect: When we demonstrate an act of kindness to another, it inspires that person to perform a similar act for someone else. In this way, our small act of kindness multiplies in ways that we cannot readily perceive. Do not think that your small act of kindness becomes lost in the negativity of the world. It is said that the positive energy that we bring to existence makes a healing difference, even if we cannot directly perceive it. (See "Further Reading" for resources on Taoism and Buddhism; see also Chopra, Dossey, and Ferrini.)

 Identify three small acts of kindness that you can offer to others this week. Practice offering this kindness without any expectation. Describe in your journal the feelings you experienced surrounding each act. In time, you will be able to extend such acts of compassion and kindness to your own daily life with greater ease.

Taoism

Cleary, T. F., Laozi, T. C., & Zhuangzi, N-H. C. (1993). *The essential Tao: An initiation into the heart of Taoism through the authentic Tao Te Ching and the inner teachings of Chaung-Tzu*. San Francisco: HarperCollins.

Lao-tzu. (1998). *Tao te ching* (S. Mitchell, Trans.). New York: Harper Perennial. (Original work, n.d.)

Weber, M. (1951). *The religion of China: Confucianism and Taoism*. Glencoe, IL: Free Press.

Buddhism

Dalai Lama. (2001). *An open heart: Practicing compassion in everyday life* (N. Vreeland, Ed.). New York: Little Brown.

Dalai Lama. (2002). *How to practice: The way to a meaningful life* (J. Hopkins, Ed. & Trans.). New York: Atrai Books.

Dalai Lama, & Cutler, H. C. (1998). *The art of happiness: A handbook for living*. New York: Riverhead Books.

Nhat Hanh, T. (1991). *Peace is every step: The path to mindfulness in everyday life*. New York: Bantam Books.

Nhat Hanh, T. (1993). *For a future to be possible: Commentaries on the five wonderful precepts*. Berkeley, CA: Parallax Press.

Nhat Hanh, T. (1995). *Zen keys: A guide to Zen practice*. New York: Doubleday.

Nhat Hanh, T. (1998). *The heart of the Buddha's teaching: Transforming suffering into peace, joy, and liberation. The four noble truths, the noble eightfold path, and other basic Buddhist teachings*. Berkeley, CA: Parallax Press.

Nhat Hanh, T., & Vo, D. M. (1987). *The miracle of mindfulness: A manual on meditation*. Boston: Beacon Press.

Healing Through Forgiveness

Chopra, D. (1993). *Ageless body, timeless mind: The quantum alternative to growing old*. New York: Harmony Books.

Ferrini, P. (1991). *The 12 steps of forgiveness: A practical manual for moving from fear to love*. Greenfield, MA: Heartways Press.

Ferrini, P. (1994). *Love without conditions: Reflections of the Christ mind*. Greenfield, MA: Heartways Press.

Weil, A. (1995). *Spontaneous healing: How to discover and enhance your body's natural ability to maintain and heal itself*. New York: Fawcett Columbine.

Mythology and the Lessons of Human Life

Campbell, J. (1959). *The masks of God*. New York: Viking Press.

Campbell, J. (1968). *The hero with a thousand faces*. Princeton, NJ: Princeton University Press.

Campbell, J. (1972). *Myths to live by: How we create ancient legends in our daily lives to release human potential*. New York: Bantam Books.

Tatge, C. (Producer). (1988). *Joseph Campbell and the power of myth: With Bill Moyers* [Videorecording]. New York: Mystic Fire Video.

Serenity Prayer and Healing Through Prayer

Dossey, L. (1993). *Healing words: The power of prayer and the practice of medicine.* San Francisco: HarperCollins.

Pietsch, W. V. (1990). *The serenity prayer book.* San Francisco: HarperCollins.

Tolson, C. L., & Koenig, H. G. (2003). *The healing power of prayer: The surprising connection between prayer and your health.* Grand Rapids, MI: Baker Books.

A

Acceptance
    anecdote, 18–22, 48–51
    identification, 22–23
    of loss, 3, 4
    of others, 22
    of the present, 71–73
Accomplishments, 26–27
Activity, 11–12
Adaptation, 3–4, 50–51
Adversity, 122–123
Advice, 155
Advocacy, 133
Analysis, 68
Anger, 77, 96
Anxiety, 64–65, 106
Appreciation, 63–64, 65, 138
Attachment, 51–53
Attacks, 41–42
Attitudes, 98
Auto accident anecdote, 48–51
Awareness, 66–69

B

Baby boomers, 100–101
Balance, 65–66, 153

Blame
    forgiveness, 38
    for illness, 34
    overcoming, 80
Breathing, 67–68
Brokenness, 58–60, 86

C

Cancer anecdote, 62–66
Car accident anecdote, 48–51
Caretaker role, 153–154
Caring, 158
Celebration, 12–14
Children, 78–79
Choices, 103–105
Chronic fatigue syndrome,
    126–131
Coincidences, 121–122
Compassion
    anecdote, 32–38
    definition, 39
    experience of, 159–160
    source of, 151–152
    toward others, 41
    toward self, 40–41
    views of, 38–40

Control
    anecdote, 94–99
    giving up, 52
    inappropriateness,
        154–155
    over others, 78–79
    realistic assessment,
        102–105
    relinquishing, 54,
        56–58
    views of, 99–101
Criticism
    examining, 24–25
    forgiveness, 42
    self-talk, 82–83
Cycles of life, 7–8

D

Death, 123–124, 141
Deficit thinking, 58–59
Dependence, 56, 129–130
Depression anecdote, 32–38
Diabetes anecdote, 94–99
Disability, 58
Disappointment, 5, 97
Drowning anecdote,
    108–115

E

Effort, 25–27, 144–145
Emotions
    communicating to
        others, 141–142
    control over, 104
    forgiveness, 45–46

    during grieving, 9–11
    healing, 139–140
    opposition to, 85–86
    release, 83–87
    repressing, 77
Envy, 19
Expectations
    attachment to, 52–53
    for others, 154
    overcoming, 71–72
    relinquishing, 55–56
    review of, 26
    revising, 49–51
    unrealistic, 96–98
experience, 53–54

F

Failure, 26–27
Faith
    acceptance, 23
    acceptance of disability,
        20
    and illness, 96, 97
Fantasizing, 95
Fear
    of death, 123–124
    insecurity, 78–79
    overcoming, 74
    for safety, 101
Fixing, 58–60
Flexibility (emotional),
    54–55
Forgiveness
    of others, 37, 44–46
    of self, 37–38, 42–44

Future, 64–65, 74

G
Giving
  anecdote, 148–152
  returns from, 159–161
  and self-pity, 87
Goals, 98
Gratitude
  demonstration, 13
  for illness, 135
  for the present, 70–71
  and self-pity, 87
Grief
  anecdote, 2–6
  permission, 8–10
  release, 85
Growth, 14, 54
Grudges, 44–45
Guilt, 42, 85

H
Happiness, 80
Healing, 124, 152
Heart attack, 76–81
Help
  appropriateness,
    152–155
  asking for, 130–131
  deserving, 133–134
  small acts, 157
Heroes, 147, 155–156
Hope, 151–152
Humiliation, 19
Humility, 133–134

I
Illness
  as gift, 125
  messages of, 131–141
  view of, 27–29
Inadequacy, 83–84
Insecurity, 78
Isolation, 19–20

J
Journeys, 121–123
Judgment, 72
Justice, 116

K
Kindness, 160–161

L
Letter writing, 10
Letting go, 4–5
Life lessons, 118–120,
  155–157
Lifestyle changes
  after illness, 128–129
  message about, 132,
    135–136
Listening, 155
Loss, 2–6
Love, 21, 141

M
Meals, 68–69
Memorials, 158–159
Mentors, 117–118, 156–157

Mindfulness training
    compassion, 40
    and negative self-talk, 83
    self-acceptance, 24–25
Mistakes
    accepting in self, 82–83
    allowing in others, 78–79
    forgiveness, 43
Motorcycle accident anecdote,
    2–6
Movement disorder anecdote,
    18–22

N
Negativity
    anecdote, 76–81
    forgiveness, 44
    mindfulness, 24–25
    moving beyond, 14–15
    self-talk, 81–83
    in speech, 73

O
Opportunities, 53–54, 112–114
Opposition, 85–86, 87

P
Pain, 67
Perfection, 36, 98
Permission, 8–10
Perseverance
    after loss, 6
    benefits, 149
    faith, 111–112

Perspective, 80–81, 103
Plans, 50–51
Positive experiences, 87–89
Positive perspective, 14–15
Presence, 62–66
Present
    appreciation, 138
    focus on, 69–70
    spiritual meaning,
        120–121
    and uncertainty, 105–106
Punishment, 86–87
Purpose, 142–145

R
Regret, 4
Rejection, 77–78
Relationships
    accepting differences,
        79–80
    after illness, 129–131
    forgiveness, 45–46
    healing, 138–139
    and life lessons,
        119–120
Release, 10–11
Resentment, 116–117
Respect, 154
Responses, 104
Responsibility
    appropriateness, 153
    choosing, 137
    relinquishing, 56–58
Rituals, 12–14

S

Safety, 101
Satisfaction, 70–71
Self-acceptance, 18–23
Self-care, 134–136
Self-image, 14–16, 123–124
Self-pity, 87
Self-talk, 81–83
Self-worth, 133
Sensations, 66–69
Silence, 68–69
Slowing down, 131–133
Small steps, 98
Speech, 73
Speech therapist anecdote,
    148–152
Spirituality
       anecdote, 108–115
       lessons, 117–121
       views, 115–117

Standards, 36, 43
Suicide, 34
Support groups, 29

T

Time, 136–138, 141–142
Today, 73–74
Trauma, 100–101

U

Uncertainty, 100–101,
    105–106

V

Validation, 20–21

W

Wisdom, 157
Worry, 63

ABOUT THE AUTHOR

Sharon Gutman, PhD, OTR/L, has been an occupational therapist for nearly 15 years and has helped people in many patient populations rebuild their lives after injury or illness. She currently teaches in the Department of Occupational Therapy at Richard Stockton College of New Jersey.